# Nursing Research for Nursing Practice

An international perspective

*Edited by*
**REBECCA BERGMAN**

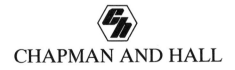

## CHAPMAN AND HALL

LONDON • NEW YORK • TOKYO • MELBOURNE • MADRAS

| UK | Chapman and Hall, 11 New Fetter Lane, London EC4P 4EE |
|---|---|
| USA | Chapman and Hall, 29 West 35th Street, New York NY10001 |
| JAPAN | Chapman and Hall Japan, Thomson Publishing Japan, Hirakawacho Nemoto Building, 7F, 1-7-11 Hirakawa-cho, Chiyoda-ku, Tokyo 102 |
| AUSTRALIA | Chapman and Hall Australia, Thomas Nelson Australia, 480 La Trobe Street, PO Box 4725, Melbourne 3000 |
| INDIA | Chapman and Hall India, R. Sheshadri, 32 Second Main Road, CIT East, Madras 600 035 |

First edition 1990

Typeset in 10/12 Times by
Leaper & Gard Ltd, Bristol
Printed in Great Britain by
T.J. Press (Padstow) Ltd, Padstow, Cornwall

ISBN 0 412 33500 X

British Library Cataloguing in Publication Data
Nursing research for nursing practice.
   1. Medicine. Nursing. Research
   I. Bergman, Rebecca
   610.73'072

ISBN 0 412 33500 X


Library of Congress Cataloging-in-Publication Data available

# Contents

# Contributors

| | |
|---|---|
| *Emilia Luigia Saporiti Angerami* | RN, PhD (University of Sao Paulo, Brazil) Professor and Dean, School of Nursing of Ribeirao Preto, University of Sao Paulo, Brazil |
| *Margaret Bennett* | RN, PhD (Monash University, Australia) Head, School of Nursing, Phillip Institute of Technology, Bundoora, Victoria, Australia |
| *Rebecca Bergman* | RN, EdD (Columbia University, USA) Professor of Nursing, Department of Nursing, Tel Aviv University, Israel |
| *Myriam Ovalle Bernal* | RN, EdD (Catholic University of America, USA) Advisor of Research, Spanish General Copuncil of Nursing, Madrid, Spain; Associate Professor, School of Nursing, University of Navarra, Spain |
| *Birgit Westphal Christensen* | RN, MPH (Nordic School of Public Health, Sweden) Acting Director, Danish Institute for Health and Nursing Research, Copenhagen, Denmark |
| *Marion R. Clark* | RN, BA (Massey University, New Zealand) Nurse Advisor, Workforce Development Group, New Zealand Department of Health, Wellington, New Zealand |
| *Laurel Archer Copp* | RN, PhD (University of Pittsburg, USA) Dean and Professor, School of Nursing, University of North Carolina at Chapel Hill, USA |

| | |
|---|---|
| *Marie Farrell* | RN, EdD (Boston University, USA)<br>Regional Officer for Nursing, Midwifery, Social Work Services, European Region, World Health Organization, Copenhagen, Denmark |
| *M. Josephine Flaherty* | RN, PhD (University of Toronto, Canada)<br>Principal Nursing Officer, National Department of Health and Welfare, Government of Canada, Ottawa, Canada |
| *Janet Heinrich* | RN, DrPH (Yale University, USA)<br>Director, Division of Extramural Programs, National Center for Nursing Research, National Institute of Health, Bethesda, USA |
| *Ada Sue Hinshaw* | RN, PhD (University of Arizona, USA)<br>Director, National Center for Nursing Research, National Institute of Health, Bethesda, USA |
| *Miriam J. Hirschfeld* | RN, DNSc (University of California, San Francisco, USA)<br>Head, Generic Baccalaureate Program, Department of Nursing, Tel Aviv University, Israel |
| *Tamar Krulik* | RN, DNSc (University of California, San Francisco, USA)<br>Head, Department of Nursing, Tel Aviv University, Israel |
| *Syringa Marshall-Burnett* | RN, MA (New York University, USA)<br>Acting Director, Advanced Nursing Education Unit, Faculty of Medical Sciences, University of the West Indies, Kingston, Jamaica |
| *Philippa J. Moore* | BSc (University of Canterbury, New Zealand)<br>Advisory Officer, Workforce Development Group, New Zealand Department of Health, Wellington, New Zealand |
| *Astrid Norberg* | RN, PhD (University of Lund, Sweden)<br>Professor of Nursing Science, Department of Advanced Nursing, University of Umeå, Sweden |

*Charlotte Searle*  RN, PhD (University of Pretoria, RSA)
Professor and Consultant of Nursing, University
of South Africa, Pretoria and Dean, Faculty of
Nursing and Medical Sciences, University of
Namibia

*Elaine Y.N. Wang*  BSc, Master of Health Administration
(University of New South Wales, Australia)
Advisory Officer, Workforce Development
Group, New Zealand Department of Health,
Wellington, New Zealand

# Preface

This book was born when Christine Birdsall, formerly Nursing Editor of Chapman and Hall Publishers, read an article titled 'Escaping from the ivory tower' (Bergman, 1986). The paper reviewed some of the nursing research carried out in Israel, situations that triggered the various studies and how the findings were utilized within the reality of Israeli society. The publisher invited the author of the article to develop this theme into a book. The scope of the original article was changed from a national to an international perspective in order to show the development and impact of nursing research in different societies within the context of their specific socio-economic-political settings.

Outstanding nurse researchers from around the world were invited to contribute chapters. They were requested to describe briefly the major aspects of health and nursing in their country and then relate in depth to an important area of nursing research with emphasis on its utilization in nursing practice and education.

Readers will make several journeys in this book, visiting countries around the globe with differing cultures and socio-political beliefs: Australia, New Zealand, South Africa, Israel, Sweden, Spain, Canada, USA, Jamaica and Brazil. They will learn how nurses in countries with limited resources focus on urgent essential problems, while others, in countries with longstanding research tradition and support are able to conduct sophisticated experimental clinical studies.

Readers will also be exposed to approaches and resources for nursing research at three organizational levels. The global dimension is represented by the research endeavours of the International Council of Nurses and the World Health Organization; the continental scope by the research programme of the European region of WHO; and the recently established USA National Center for Nursing Research provides a country-wide perspective.

An additional cardinal objective of the book is to offer the reader a variety of research topics with chapters in each of the areas of education, clinical practice, nursing administration and legislation. The authors were requested to select a topic within their field of expertise. The papers from

Jamaica and Canada report research on education of nurses for primary health and on preparation of nurse researchers respectively. Most of the clinical practice chapters include reference to related educational and administrative aspects but focus primarily on nursing interventions. They include the subjects of pain (USA), dementia (Sweden) and chronic illness (Israel). Nursing administration research includes studies on patient dependency (Australia) and manpower (New Zealand). The chapters from Brazil (primary health care), Spain (nursing education and practice systems) and South Africa (status of nursing as a profession) highlight the relationship between sociopolitical factors, legislation and nursing research. The final chapter looks to the future priorities for nursing research, based on a short review of the major trends over the past half century.

This group of international authors invites the readers to join them on this round-the-world, many-faceted journey of nursing research. Hopefully, the experience will lead to greater international awareness and exchange resulting in enhanced co-operation in research, practice and education.

Rebecca Bergman

## REFERENCE

Bergman, R. (Oct 8, 1986) Escaping from the ivory tower. *Nurs. Times*, **82**, 58–60.

# CHAPTER ONE

# All the world's a stage: the role of international organizations in nursing research

*Rebecca Bergman*

Many international bodies are playing an important role in nursing research. Two such organizations are the World Health Organization (WHO) and the International Council of Nurses (ICN).

Research, although not the major mission of either organization, is included in their programmes. Other organizations at the global level occasionally conduct nursing-related research. Among these are the League of Red Cross Societies (LORCS), the United Nations International Childrens' Emergency Fund (UNICEF) and the International Council of Midwives (ICM). The more recently established international specialty nursing organizations such as those of oncological, critical care, or geriatric nursing contribute to the dissemination of research findings through their conferences and literature. Regional organizations, both nursing (e.g. Scandinavian Nurses' Organization) or intergovernmental (European Economic Council) often support nursing research and conduct surveys or evaluative studies.

Some nursing research is funded by private foundations. An example of this is the Kellogg Foundation which introduced a fellowship programme in 1987 that includes several research projects in the field of nursing. An Israeli fellow is conducting a three-year research-practice programme to improve the care of chronically ill children at home. A USA fellow is examining perceptions of management, including nursing, in several countries around the world (Krulik, 1988).

A further dimension of international nursing research is cross-national nursing study initiated and conducted by individuals or teams in several countries using the same tools and collating the findings for a comprehensive report. For example, faculty of the University of California San Francisco are co-operating with researchers in several countries. One study, together with Chinese nurses, focuses on professional socialization of the first baccalaureate nursing students in the People's Republic of China. A USA–Australian research is concerned with aspects of euthanasia. A seven-country study on the ethics of force-feeding includes teams in Sweden, Finland, Israel, USA, Japan, China and Australia (Davis, 1988).

This chapter will focus on two major organizations, ICN and WHO. It will present their position statements in relation to nursing research and briefly discuss some of their studies.

### THE INTERNATIONAL COUNCIL OF NURSES

ICN was established in 1899, by representatives of seven nursing organizations. By 1989 membership had increased to 101 national nurses' associations representing about 1 100 000 nurses (Holleran, 1989).

In 1977, the Council of National Representatives approved the following definition of nursing research:

'The International Council of Nurses is convinced of the importance of nursing research as a major contribution to meeting the health and welfare needs of people. The continuous and rapid scientific developments in a changing world highlight the need for research as a means of identifying new knowledge, improving professional education and practice and effectively utilizing resources.

'ICN believes that nursing research should be socially relevant. It should look to the future while drawing on the past and being concerned with the present.

'Nursing research should include both that which relates to a total research plan and that which may be undertaken independently. In nursing research available resources of different levels of sophistication should be utilized and research should comply with accepted ethical standards. Research findings should be widely disseminated and their utilization and implementation encouraged when appropriate.

'ICN believes that nurses should initiate and carry out research in areas specific to nursing and collaborate with related professions in research on other aspects of health. Nursing research should involve nurses practising in the area under study.

National nurses associations are urged to promote the development and utilization of nursing research in co-operation with other interested groups.'

Together with the 1977 definition, the role of the associations was spelled out:

'Nurses associations can contribute to the development and the quality of nursing education and nursing service by promoting nursing research in their countries. The human and material resources as well as the scope of involvement in this effort vary from country to country. Therefore the following guidelines are presented as possible avenues for action which need to be adapted to the local scene by the nurses associations.

## Organizational framework

The establishment of a nursing research group within the association can provide a basis for determining association policy and action on nursing research. Such a group may take various forms such as a research committee, a section of nurse researchers, a research foundation.

This group may include nurse researchers, nurses in the various fields of nursing service and nursing education and other qualified persons who can enrich the group.

## Functions

*Education.* The association should promote an appreciation and understanding of research and the preparation of nurse researchers. Inclusion of a research component in basic and post-basic nursing education programmes, workshops, study days and other media may contribute to the achievement of this aim.

*Co-ordination.* The association should explore and develop channels for co-ordination and co-operation with other groups concerned with nursing and health-related research such as government agencies, professional organizations, educational institutions, research institutes, foundations and other non-governmental agencies.

*Survey.* In co-operation with other groups, the association should survey the scope and direction of completed and on-going research. This overview could be used to identify gaps and overlaps in order to set priorities for future projects.

*Master plan.* The association may participate in the development of a long-term master plan which could serve as a guide to researchers in the selection of projects and for the allocation of resources. However, such a master plan should not inhibit creative interests and efforts that fall outside the plan.

*Facilitation.* The association may facilitate research among its members by identifying and/or providing, where possible, guidance, consultation, funds and other resources. A forum for discussion of on-going research may offer guidance and encouragement to researchers. The association may encourage the creation or development of a system of information concerning completed nursing research in that country.

*Dissemination.* The association should encourage the distribution of research findings and implementation of the recommendations when appropriate.'

Many associations requested that ICN identify nursing research resources. Accordingly, in 1977 the ICN Board decided to gather infor-mation on available research units. A nursing unit was defined as one which 'is specifically recognized for teaching research methodology: collecting information about research related to nursing and nurses; conducting research for the purpose of improving nursing practice and the quality of patient/client care; and expanding knowledge for the develop-ment and testing of nursing theories.' A list of units was distributed in 1979 and included information on the structure of the units, their functions and activities, variables influencing their activities, the impact of their research and the topics of major studies. Update of information on research units continues to be assembled, compiled and distributed periodically.

The Board felt that ICN's role and responsibilities in nursing research needed clarification. Such a statement was prepared and it states:

'The main elements of ICN's role in relation to research are: – facilitation, e.g. promoting research, preparing guidelines, organizing a research program during ICN congresses and other such activities; and – collabor-ation with national and international organizations in regard to the conduct of nursing and other relevant research, the sharing of information and the use of research results.

National nurses associations are urged to promote the development and utilization of nursing research in co-operation with other interested groups.'

As the national associations increased their involvement in research, they requested more direction from ICN. In 1985, ICN published a set of guidelines for nursing research. They include five sections and two appen-dices which are summarized below.

1.  Appraisal of the organizational climate for research – such as the values towards research, awareness, commitment, time used for research activities, formal and informal rewards, availability of research grants, 'critical mass' of researchers, etc.
2.  Organization – the setting; lines of relationships between the research

endeavours and the parent organization; activities additional to the conduct of research such as courses, workshops, disseminating findings, consultation; review by advisory or steering committees, peers or external readers.

3. Resources – such as the number and qualification of human resources, mentorships of experienced researchers to neophytes, communality among the researchers; material resources including space, equipment, library, computer, finances.
4. Research programme – core research programme v. separate studies, generation of research questions, relevance of research to health needs, ethical considerations and evaluation of the research.
5. Role of national nurses associations (1977) as reported above.

The appendices provide guidelines for the development of a research proposal and how to obtain the resources needed to support it.

At this time there was felt a need to review and update the 1977 definition of nursing research. In 1987 a new definition was approved by the Council of National Representatives (CNR).

*Preamble.* 'The future of nursing practice and ultimately the future of health care depends on nursing research designed to constantly generate an up-to-date organized body of nursing knowledge.

'Nursing, as an integral part of the health care system, encompasses the promotion of health, prevention of illness and care of the physically ill, mentally ill and disabled people of all ages, in all health care and other community settings. Within this broad spectrum of health care, the phenomena of particular concern to nurses are individual, family and group responses to actual or potential health problems. These human responses range from health-restoring reactions to an individual episode of illness to the development of policy in promoting the long-term health of a population. Nursing research thus spans a wide range of investigation areas.

*Nursing research.* 'Nursing research focuses on developing knowledge of the care of persons in health and illness. It is directed toward understanding the fundamental genetic, physiological, social, behavioural and environmental mechanisms that affect the ability of individuals and families to maintain or enhance optimum function and minimize the negative effects of illness.

'Nursing research also emphasizes the generation of knowledge of policies and systems that effectively and efficiently deliver nursing care; the profession and its historical development; ethical guidelines for the delivery of nursing services; and systems that effectively and efficiently prepare nurses to fulfil the profession's current and future social mandate.'

'In addition, principal investigators who are nurses often conduct scientific inquiry into the cause, diagnosis and prevention of diseases, the promotion of health, the processes of human growth and development and the biological effects of environmental contaminants. These foci, however, are not unique to nursing.'

Although ICN to date has not directly undertaken research projects, its contribution to nursing research has been considerable through the definition of nursing research, clarification of roles of the National Association and of ICN, the directory of research centres and the guidelines. These documents have been particularly helpful to younger and smaller nursing associations that do not have the experience and resources of the more established groups.

### WORLD HEALTH ORGANIZATION (WHO)

WHO is a specialized agency of the United Nations with primary responsibility for international health matters and public health. The organization was created in 1948, and presently has 166 countries in membership.

WHO promotes the development of comprehensive health services, the prevention and control of diseases, the improvement of environmental conditions, the development of health manpower, the co-ordination and development of health services, research and the planning and implementation of health programmes. The present major goal of WHO, based on the Declaration of Alma-Ata in 1978, is the attainment of 'Health for All by the Year 2000' with emphasis on the development of Primary Health Care (PHC).

The two major divisions, Development of Health Manpower and Development of Health Services, are instrumental in promoting nursing research. They encourage nursing research, particularly program evaluation at the operation level. WHO also carries out some research initiated by Geneva headquarters or by the regional offices.

In the last decade, WHO focused on PHC research using an interdisciplinary approach. The WHO Advisory Committee on Medical Research (WHO, 1988) states that research 'should be both oriented towards and justified by the contribution it can make to improve health systems.' It should include four major elements (given below), all of which have implications for nursing.

1. *The health care system*, including: health care needs; organization for delivery of care; management of health care organizations; cost factors; quality of care provided; and roles of consumers.
2. *Health manpower development*, including: manpower planning to meet health systems needs; manpower mix and distribution; determination

of manpower competencies; planning, organizing, implementing and evaluating basic and continuing educational programmes for health workers; teamwork; and manpower management (employment, incentives, career schemes, living and working conditions, etc.)

3. *Organizational factors,* including: characteristics of health service and health personnel education institutions; characteristics of professional health worker organizations or unions (e.g. orientation, values, etc.); and community development and health involvement schemes

4. *Social/cultural, demographic factors,* including: resources available for health care; community aspirations, behaviours and values related to health; political philosophy as it influences health services; and demographic features

The report emphasizes that research projects will have to be formulated and pursued in relation to realistic field settings and that every effort should be made to ensure utilization of the findings. They define research as a 'systematic inquiry designed to produce new insights into the problems that may be global, international, national, individual, cellular or molecular in nature'. In relation to methodology they state that 'while rigidly controlled, statistically-oriented hypothesis testing should not be excluded, the problems in this field require inquiry methods that are equally rigorous but not experimental. Thus descriptive studies, case studies and sample surveys may all contribute important knowledge'. They therefore recommend both the conventional approach with emphasis on scientific objectivity, as well as the naturalistic approach with emphasis on social phenomena using qualitative methods.

Three studies, initiated by the Geneva office, will illustrate the scope and variety of such projects.

The WHO multinational study of the International migration of physicians and nurses (Mejia, Pizuki and Royston, 1979) was based on an extensive review of the literature, data gathered by questionnaire on 137 countries, and an in-depth sample of 40 countries that have considerable migration of health personnel.

The objectives of the study were:

1. To analyse the characteristics of the migrants; dimensions, directions, determinants and consequences of the flow; and
2. To suggest measures to modify the migration in desired ways.

It was hoped that this information could assist national administrations in developing measures to alleviate the problems and to develop long-term manpower policies.

Major findings of this project on nursing include:

'On average, each year some 15 000 nurses left their country. In terms of the total number of nurses, this was less than 0.5%. It was estimated that not more than 5% of the world's nurses are outside of their country of origin or training. The chief recipients of foreign nurses were the USA, UK, Canada and West Germany. The chief donors of nurses were the Philippines, the UK and Australia. The developed countries of the world received 92% of the migrant nurses but also supplied 60% of them. Very little is known about the characteristics of migrant nurses as a whole. In the UK they tended to fill the gaps such as in psychiatric hospitals.

'The international migration is the result of push and pull factors. The poorer the country, the greater is likely to be its loss relative to domestic stock. Income differentials may play a role in nurse migration. Policies and practices in the recipient countries with regard to migration are more effective in determining the volume and direction of migration than are policies and practices of the donor country. International agreements promoting international recognition of nursing qualifications facilitate and possibly encourage migration.'

This study provided the first available comprehensive picture of nurse migration. It revealed that the global scope of nurse migration was not a severe problem, but did require national intervention in specific countries.

A second example of a WHO nursing study examined the utilization and training of traditional birth attendants (Mangay-Maglacas and Pizurki, 1981). As traditional birth attendants (TBA) provide much of the basic health care for rural populations in many developing countries, the authors felt that the 'experience in one country with TBA training, supervision, evaluation and practices can be of great value and interest to others', particularly as 'In many countries several decades will pass before national resources will be sufficient to allow for the development of an adequate number of qualified staff.' Their recommendations include:

'Health professionals should make efforts to overcome their resistance to accepting TBAs as legitimate health workers ...
Efforts should be made to overcome the TBAs resistance to being controlled in any way by staff of the health system ...
TBAs should be closely and regularly supervised in order to ensure that they are performing their work as they were taught ...
Efforts should be made to provide a sufficient number of trainers and supervisors to ensure that they are qualified to train and supervise TBAs ...
Training programmes for TBAs should be designed to take into account the major health and health-related problems of the community concerned, the cultural values of the community, and the characteristics of the TBAs, particularly their age, level of general education

and the manner in which they communicate with members of the community ...
Efforts should be made to develop an adequate referral system.'

The third illustration of WHO nursing research is a survey of post-basic training programmes for nurse educators and managers (Maillart and Mangay-Maglacas, 1983). The major objective was 'to clarify the role of the post-basic programmes and their components in the process of curriculum change in preparation of nurse educators and managers'. Data was collected by means of a comprehensive mailed questionnaire from 100 schools in 43 countries in all six WHO regions.
Major conclusions include:

1. Curriculum revision was taking place in more than three-quarters of the schools. They emphasized student involvement in health services, independent study, programme flexibility;
2. The major change agent was often the educational director, with support of needed resources;
3. Attachment of a programme to hospital services often impeded curriculum revision, particularly in the direction of primary health care;
4. Graduates of these programmes required more skill development in planning, developing and implementing management and educational programs;
5. Educator or manager positions did not receive sufficient financial remuneration or social recognition;
6. Co-ordination with other professions and among schools in the same country needed to be enriched;
7. Programme awards in such programmes were changing from certificates to degrees, with the trend to master degrees;
8. Follow-up studies of graduates to evaluate the relevancy of the programmes were strongly recommended.

These three examples illustrate the variety of WHO nursing research.
In addition to WHO studies, the organization encourages and occasionally funds nursing and interdisciplinary research projects of national teams and individuals.
The prime contribution to nursing research by these major international organizations is in their global perspective. Not less important is the support which they provide to nursing researchers through guidelines, identification of research questions, encouragement and recognition of researchers and dissemination of their work through publication.
The growing recognition of the importance of cross-fertilization of nursing research between countries has created the need for more worldwide research. Nurses and nursing groups are reaching out to each other

across borders and between cultures. International agencies, such as ICN and WHO, can serve as communication hubs and support systems to these international endeavours.

## REFERENCES

Davis, A. (1988) personal communication.

Holleran, C. (1989) personal communication.

Krulik, T. (1988) personal communication.

Maillart, V. and Mangay-Maglacas, A. (1983) *Report on a Survey of Post-basic Training Programmes for Nurse Teachers (Educators) and Administrators (Managers).* World Health Organization, Geneva.

Mangay-Maglacas, A. and Pizurki, H. (1981) The traditional birth attendant in seven countries: Case studies in utilization and training. *Public Health Papers,* no. 75, World Health Organization, Geneva.

Mejia, A., Pizurki, H. and Royston, E. (1979) *Physician and Nurse Migration.* World Health Organization, Geneva.

WHO (1988) 'Advisory Committee on Medical Research'. Internal document, World Health Organization, Geneva.

# CHAPTER TWO

# Coming of age: nursing research in Europe

*Marie Farrell and Birgit Westphal Christensen*

## INTRODUCTION

Nursing research in Europe has undergone profound change in the past ten years. The number and variety of publications, projects, studies, and courses have grown at a considerable rate. Community and hospital services have developed research elements as part of overall evaluation, and schools and university programmes include research as part of the curriculum.

The integration of quality assurance elements into the health care system has highlighted the need for specificity and underscores the concern for documentation and monitoring of care in measurable terms. Courses in nursing theory building, statistics, computer technology and research methods are popular and demand for World Health Organization (WHO) collaboration in these areas is growing.

This groundswell of interest and activity might be understood by considering the change process which has been under way in nursing research in the European Region of WHO between 1970 and 1988; these developments set the stage for the present and future emphases which will occupy the efforts of nurses in the years to 2000.

## BACKGROUND

Nursing research in Europe has its origins with Florence Nightingale who reminded nurses that 'merely looking at the sick is not observing'. Observation remains a basic tool used in nursing research, and is one of the first and last subjects taught to students; in this sense, European nurses are and have always been researchers, and they share many of the methods used by other scientists in their daily practice.

Nursing is work which finds meaning in action; this action is to provide a service rather than to provide a product for people. Because people are dynamic, the actions required by nurses are dynamic, and require continual study and change. For this reason, nursing research is the foundation of care and becomes outdated the day the nurse stops changing her practice.

Historically, for many, European nursing was synonymous with individual patient care. Traditionally, nurses were competent, efficient and seen more often in the workplace applying knowledge gained somewhere else rather than presenting themselves as applied scientists gathering data in the field. The results of research were introduced into the student's curriculum and into the clinical settings in which nurses worked; but the emphasis was not on the research process itself, but on the changes made to improve the situation for the patient. Emphasis was on the activities which had to be completed, with less discussion on the reasons why changes were being made or on why nurses were taking on another activity.

Implicitly, assumptions were made that the new tasks were in keeping with the accepted role of the nurse, which were in turn part of the functions of the nurse as provider of care, as teacher, and counsellor. No nurse would consider using techniques that were outdated, or of giving information which was no longer considered valid. However, after the Second World War, economic, social and political factors affected the availability of personnel and resources, and 'coverage', rather than use of the latest research findings, was the major preoccupation. The concern was to provide basic care with extremely limited resources. During these years, the European Economic Community (EEC) paid more attention to the standardization of nursing education than to the development of nursing research.

In the 1960s and 1970s the European Economic Commission discussions and directives focused on the relative mobility of nurses rather than on the nature of their practice and care of people. The Dahrendorf Hearing in 1973 placed emphasis on the acceptance of professional diplomas and stressed the competence of the practitioner (Ashworth, Bjørn, Déchanoz *et al.*, 1987).

By the mid-1970s, nurses, like other health providers, began to experience profound changes from within and without the disciplines. An explosion of knowledge occurred; new professions were developing and the sheer workload put on nurses was well beyond the resources available to them or to the organizations in which they worked. Nurses were expected to provide discharge teaching, work with communities, serve as advocates of the family, implement family planning programmes, and provide complete antepartum teaching courses, using increasingly complex audiovisual materials. At this point, the use of computer technology was just over the horizon.

Professional and public awareness was drawn to the uneven distribution, rising costs and uncertain outcomes of the health services. Nursing services cost a great deal of money and nurses constituted a very large segment of the health care industry. Yet little was known about the way nurses cared for people, the decisions they made and the effects of their decision-making on health outcomes (Ashworth, Bjørn, Déchanoz *et al.*, 1987).

Nurses began to look at the tasks they were carrying out, and began to question the legitimacy of some of the tasks seen against their developing ideas of what nursing practice was really all about. They also realized that the needs of the person dictated their system of care, not the disease process diagnosed by the physician or the mandates of the hospital. Nurses began to separate their nursing role from the medical role, and became interested in their beliefs about what they did as differentiated from the contribution of other health workers. Nursing as an applied discipline, with its own theories and ways of thinking began to take shape, and those in practice began to talk about the way they made decisions about patient care. Nurses began to identify the steps in their decision-making process, and defined their scope to include not only individuals, but families, groups and communities as well.

While nurse leaders in Europe called for research-based knowledge about nursing, they realized that few qualified researchers were available to carry out the required work. They also realized that funding research required a track record founded on sound traditions of research which had not yet been built for nursing in the region.

The relationship between the psychological and social aspects of living and the health of the person was well accepted in nursing as fundamental to practice, and some had begun to study how they could enhance people's chances for better mental and physical wellbeing.

## NURSING IN WHO: THE 1970s

Until the early 1970s, nursing in the Regional Office for Europe of the World Health Organization consisted of activities to improve nursing education and services, using the traditional approaches of meetings, reports and fellowships. In 1974, a position paper on nursing was written (Hall, 1979) which stressed the broad range of nursing behaviours currently accepted as part of the nurse's functions. It also underscored the view that nursing is a research-based science which uses knowledge and techniques from the physical, social, mental and biological sciences and from the humanities.

During this time the Regional Office reoriented its nursing programme and stressed the decision-making process, called the nursing process, and included functions such as documenting care and carrying out research. The shift from nursing as a series of discrete tasks to viewing it as a person-centred caring process served as the focal point about which a major nursing research study was launched in the WHO Regional Office for

Europe. Parenthetically, it should be noted that all of these actions were taken before the 1978 Alma-Ata Declaration which emphasized primary health care, and many of the elements were already under study by nurses in Europe and by the Nursing unit of the Regional Office. The pivotal role of primary health care and the need for a community focus was emphasized in WHO as early as 1974, and several developments occurred in research in the European Region. The Conference of European Nurse Researchers has been held each year since 1979, and selected university and institute programmes have developed in the Region (First Conference of European Nurse Researchers, 1979; Lorensen, 1980; Lanara and Raya, 1981; Lerheim 1982).

### WHO's APPROACH TO RESEARCH IN NURSING

## Technical elements

By the end of the 1970s, the Nursing unit of the Regional Office was in its fifth general programming cycle (Fifth General Programme of Work) which was structured around the major nursing research initiative. The emphasis was to be on the caring process, the core content of nursing practice. Workshops were held which showed nurses how to record their actions, and to develop records which documented their observations, assessment, actions and evaluations of people's needs for nursing care (Prophit, 1980). While nurses in some parts of Europe considered documentation as part of their daily practice, others did not, and hospitals and other health care professionals were not used to this element of care. In fact, some providers disliked this element and felt threatened when nurses expressed interest in documentation. Yet, a written record was the basis for evaluation, research and the development of standards of practice – key issues for the future of nursing in Europe.

At this time the Regional Office used the European Advisory Committee on Medical Research (EACMR) as its major vehicle for monitoring and reviewing research in the Region. The nursing multinational study was launched, with reviews carried out by this body. No unified Regional Office research strategy had yet been developed, and no nurse had yet been appointed to this group.

## Operational aspects

Before the research effort could be launched, a series of negotiations had to be held with governments and authorities at national and regional levels. Funds were required to staff at least the programme managers' posts, and the participation of several hundred people in the 11 countries was required. Thus, the Fifth and Sixth General Programmes of Work also included creating a regional network of links through a series of collaborating centres which would serve as the national centres for teaching, collection of data and development of research activities. Secondary centres (called Type I and Type II Centres) were also used to teach the decision-making process in nursing, and to reinforce nursing research activities in the country.

The participants in the 11 countries held workshops, seminars and on-site experiences in interviewing patients, recording data, developing data collection instruments and using coding procedures during data collection. The nurse programme managers developed further their computer literacy skills, learned how to read computer printouts, and how to assess their data collection tools for validity, reliability, and other characteristics. The same group of 11 managers were also the writers of this first international collaborative study on nursing which constituted the activities of the Fifth and Sixth General Programme of Work in WHO in nursing (Ashworth, Bjørn, Déchanoz *et al.*, 1987).

## Public relations aspects

The challenges to the Regional Office and the programme managers during the seven years of the multinational study were many. One of the most critical was obtaining and maintaining the financial support for the many activities which were part of the learning required. Two countries dropped out (leaving 11 in the final count) partly because of funding expectations of the donors, and partly because of the inability to maintain the momentum and support for teaching and learning required. Clearly, considerable faith in the process was required, and nurses in leadership positions demonstrated remarkable ability in arguing the case for research in Europe in general, and in the work of the remaining 11 countries in particular (Nursing Care: Summary of a European Study, 1987).

### DEVELOPING A REGIONAL STRATEGY FOR HEALTH

While these efforts were under way, the Regional Office for Europe with its 32 member countries of Europe (Member States), adopted specific, measurable expectations for the Region. After several drafts involving hundreds of professionals, lay people and volunteer groups in Europe, 38 targets for health were approved by the WHO Regional Committee in 1984. The Regional Committee is a kind of European parliament for health where delegates from the Member States meet each year and evaluate progress made towards reaching the agreed-upon targets. Mechanisms have since been established to report changes in indicators of progress made, and the programming format and organization of the Regional Office has been changed to facilitate meeting the targets.

## A HEALTH-FOR-ALL RESEARCH POLICY

The targets served as the basis on which the framework for a Regional Office plan of priority research for health for all was developed. Further, the plan developed Target 32 which calls for formulation of research strategies to stimulate investigation and to improve the use of available knowledge in the countries. Specifically, Target 32 states, 'Before 1990, all Member States should have formulated research strategies to stimulate investigations which improve the application and expansion of knowledge needed to support their health for all development' (Targets for Health for All, 1985).

The name of the European Advisory Committee on Medical Research was changed to the European Advisory Committee on Health Research, and a standing committee on research called the European Research Advisory Group was formed in the Regional Office to review proposed research projects from their inception (particularly if the planned study was at a predetermined level of funding) and to put forward to the Regional Programme Committee concrete proposals for changes or adaptations required. Nursing in the Regional Office has been and is still a member of this standing committee.

The objectives of the health-for-all research policy are to:

1. specify the criteria for setting research priorities;
2. establish goals and set priorities;
3. identify neglected areas of research;
4. identify the education, training and manpower needs resulting from the suggested priorities;
5. guarantee the national and intellectual prerequisites for research;
6. allocate resources according to the goals and priorities; and
7. facilitate the use of research findings (Research Policy for Health for All, 1987).

The implications for nursing from this European policy are clear. 'Nursing has to broaden its scope, and fundamental changes are needed at all levels of nursing practice, education, management and research. [This is necessary to] ensure that priority needs of populations are met and that nursing has full participation in policy making and administration of health care' (Van der Arend, 1986).

Currently, nursing research in Europe is under way in many areas of education and practice, and several research studies are looking at critical areas of investigation. For example, in Denmark nurses are developing ways of caring for elderly women discharged early from hospital after hip replacement surgery. This group of elderly is growing in number and requires careful planning to ensure optimum care at a cost the country can afford. Alternative scenarios are being explored so that early discharge does not result in high recidivism rates and physical and emotional setbacks.

Much of nursing research focuses on the process of care; few studies have identified outcome measures for study. Urgently needed are studies which compare the relative merits of alternative approaches, particularly in the home, and which assess the factors which account for acceptable and cost-effective nursing interventions. Given the short hospital stay, pre- and post-hospital strategies for teaching and rehabilitation are essential and the research which assesses these elements is critical.

Currently, some types of research can be identified which appear repeatedly in the literature. They fall into the following five areas:

1.  health behaviour and lifestyle assessment;
2.  evaluation of models of promotive health care;
3.  social actions/community development/community participation;
4.  quality of care; and
5.  care of the ageing.

Using the adopted WHO framework for research for health for all, one can easily identify what is available as findings and what is needed. The plan can also be used as a basis for formulating a plan for investigating the needed knowledge.

Questions such as the following can be raised:

How do midwives' perceptions of their role differ from those of their clients and from those of health officials?

How do care practices of nurses differ from those expected in WHO descriptions?

What factors have affected the advance of nursing practice in European settings (such as awareness of the women's movement; availability of research findings; presence of a university programme in nursing; contact with international groups, etc.)?

What is the sensitivity of nurses to environmental health issues? For those communities where nurses are actively involved, what factors are related to a given level of involvement?

## EDUCATION FOR NURSING RESEARCH

A well done piece of nursing research demands the integration of many areas of knowledge, use of skills, an appreciation of the ethics involved, and the ability for communicating results to others. Researchers must be able to identify concepts, constructs, and theories. They must be able to apply statistical concepts, have some knowledge of measurement, be familiar with library resources, and be computer literate. They need to know how to use the skills of a statistician, librarian, content expert, and an editor.

While the WHO research strategy offers some guidelines, a researcher in many ways marches to the beat of a different drummer. Creativity, divergent thinking, and an active role in nursing practice are essential elements necessary to ask the important questions.

Where does one learn these skills? How does one learn how to work with the disciplines which contribute to the final product? One learns the skills by studying in the places where the experts are located, and by working with them to develop the thinking essential to research. The place of study may be a university, an institute, a university teaching medical centre, or an international organization. Researchers may have to use several places to obtain the right education and to learn from the right people. The emphasis should be on what it is one needs to learn, and on who can help one learn what is needed. The arguments on who should have access to a university teaching centre have become parochial and irrelevant.

Research is a complex, expensive and time-consuming activity. Nurses cannot afford to compartmentalize themselves, work alone, and to use only nurses as resources. They must acknowledge and enter into active partnership with those who have the expertise they do not possess. Mechanisms must be established to enable them to have the access they need to address the pressing issues which the targets suggest.

Experiences of the Regional Office for Europe between 1970 and 1988 have shown that nurses in Europe are capable, able and ready to participate actively in contributing to the body of knowledge required to change the health of people. Governments have urged nurses in Europe to become involved, and have provided support and funds for nursing research activities. Posts in nursing research have been established in ministries of health, in hospitals and community health centres. Nursing research at the university level is developing at a rapid rate, and international exchanges and forums are now considered part of the 'things nurse researchers do'. Peer review, publishing research results, and preparing proposals to fund projects and apply research findings are now common events in the Region. These events will be repeated and amplified in the years before the turn of the century. Without question nursing research has come of age in Europe and nurses are expected to make significant contributions to health care in the years to 2000. In conclusion, nursing in Europe shares the conviction of T.S. Kuhn who notes: '[People] whose research is based on shared paradigms are committed to the same rules and standards for practice. That commitment and the apparent consensus it produces are prerequisites for normal science, i.e. for the genesis and continuation of a particular research tradition' (Kuhn, 1970).

## REFERENCES

Ashworth, P., Bjørn, A., Déchanoz, G. *et al.* (1987) *People's needs for nursing care: a European study.* WHO Regional Office for Europe, Copenhagen.

*First Conference of European Nurse Researchers* (1979) National Hospital Institute of the Netherlands.

Hall, D. (1979) *Position paper on nursing.* WHO Regional Office for Europe, Copenhagen.

Kuhn, T.S. (1970) *The Structure of Scientific Revolutions.* University of Chicago Press, Illinois.

Lanara, V.A. and Raya, A.C. (eds) (1981) *Third Conference of European Nurse Researchers.* Hellenic National Graduate Nurses Association, Athens.

Lerheim, K. (ed.) (1982) *Fourth Conference of European Nurse Researchers.* Norwegian Nurses Association, Oslo.

Lorensen, M. (ed.) (1980) *Second Conference of European Nurse Researchers.* Danish Nurses Organization, Copenhagen.

*Nursing care: summary of a European study* (1987) WHO Regional Office for Europe, Copenhagen.

Prophit, P. (1980) *The needs for nursing care in selected elderly and elective surgery patient/client groups: a multinational European study.* WHO Regional Office for Europe, Copenhagen (unpublished document).

*Research policy for health for all* (1987) WHO Regional Office for Europe, Copenhagen.

*Targets for health for all* (1985) WHO Regional Office for Europe, Copenhagen.

Van der Arend, A. (1986) Ethical issues in nursing: HFA2000 and primary health care perspective, in *Proceedings of the Ninth Meeting of the Workgroup of European Nurse Nurse Researchers, Helsinki, 12–15 August, 1986.*

# CHAPTER THREE

# New initiatives in nursing research: a national perspective

## *Ada Sue Hinshaw and Janet Heinrich*

Studies of patient care were initiated by Florence Nightingale in her efforts to improve the care which soldiers received during the Crimean War in the 1800s (Cohen, 1984). Mortality was linked to specific practices and environmental factors that were remedied through nursing interventions. The birth of modern nursing was part of a larger scientific and social movement that incorporated new knowledge about bacteria, clean water, and sanitation with humane efforts to reduce unnecessary pain, suffering and death.

Today, nurses constitute the largest category of health care worker in nearly every country, bearing major responsibility for essential health care services based on scientifically sound and socially acceptable methods and technology (WHO, 1986). Nurses involved in providing essential services, be they preventive, therapeutic for acute or long-term care problems, rehabilitative or managerial, must monitor, observe, and analyse the health conditions and services in particular populations. The nurse is in a pivotal role to define health problems, understand formal and informal systems of care and to ask the difficult questions that research needs to address to improve health care.

In 1977, the World Health Organization launched the 'Health for All' movement. The resolution adopted by the 30th World Health Assemblies stated: 'A main social target of governments and the World Health Organization in the coming decades should be the attainment by all the citizens of the world by the year 2000 of the level of health that will permit them to lead a socially and economically productive life' (WHO, 1978). This resolution was reaffirmed and amplified by the Declaration of Alma-Alta which specified the essential components of primary health care as follows: '... education concerning prevailing health problems and the methods of preventing and controlling them; promotion of food supply and proper nutrition; an adequate supply of safe water and basic sanitation;

maternal and child health care, including family planning; immunization against the major infectious diseases; prevention and control of local and endemic diseases; appropriate treatment of common diseases and injuries; and provision of essential drugs' (WHO, 1978)' Efforts in the last decade have focused on mobilizing governments, private and voluntary organizations, and international economic and health care groups to revise priorities to focus on the implementation of strategies for 'Health for All.' Nurses are recognized as a major factor in the success of this movement (WHO, 1978). However, nursing research has had a limited role in the international arena in addressing common health problems that are major obstacles to achieving our common health goals.

The most prevalent health problems in developing countries are common infectious and parasitic diseases, especially diarrhoea, and respiratory infections. These problems are exacerbated by widespread early childhood malnutrition and impose the heaviest burden upon infants, young children, and child-bearing women. (Evans, Hall and Warford, 1981). The consequences of diphtheria, pertussis, tetanus, measles, poliomyelitis and tuberculosis are underestimated. They are thought to cause some five million deaths among children under 5 years, while blinding, crippling or otherwise permanently disabling an additional five million.

In industrialized countries, cardiovascular diseases, cancer and stroke are the major killers. There is a noticeable trend towards a decrease in the mortality from cardiovascular diseases due to a reduction in mortality from stroke, rheumatic heart disease and hypertensive diseases. With the increasing control of infections and nutritional diseases, cancer is rapidly becoming a major cause of morbidity and mortality in developing countries and thus a heavy burden on health care systems throughout the world. HIV infection and AIDS is fast becoming a major killer in both the industrialized and developing countries, with no cure in the foreseeable future. There have been few successful efforts to reduce these major causes of mortality, much of which should be preventable.

There is a growing consensus that the family, through its structures and functions, not only influences the health and disease pattern of the individual and the community, but is also a logical unit for self reliance in health care and a channel for the improved delivery of health services. However, the relationship between health in the family, family organization, functioning and attitudes, and affecting the quality of family life is not well established. The mother is usually the family's first health care worker, but women often have no access to information and technology, income or education. The supporting mechanisms that the family has provided for its members in the past are eroding because of economic and social pressures far beyond its control, and this is profoundly effecting the health of families and especially the health of mothers and children.

Nurses are one of the major care providers in developing and industrialized countries available to combat the numerous national and international health crises. They are particularly involved with the care of mothers, infants, the elderly and families. Often in rural areas, basic primary health care is provided by nurses and nurse practitioners. Accurate information is needed to guide the practice of nurses as they assist individuals and provide health care. Information to guide nurses in addressing these common health problems must come from research and scientific study.

## EXCELLENCE IN SCIENCE

A commitment to excellence in developing the knowledge base or science needed to guide professional practice forms the cornerstone for the establishment of the National Center for Nursing Research (NCNR). The nursing profession has been consistently mindful of the criteria of excellence in building and testing the knowledge base required for the profession. Attention to excellence will result in accurate and reliable information needed to provide effective as well as efficient nursing care.

Excellence in science includes several characteristics; depth in the knowledge base and studies which are on the 'cutting edge' of knowledge frontiers (Hinshaw, Heinrich and Bloch, 1989). Depth in the knowledge base refers to a series of studies in the same or common areas of investigation which provide evidence of similar results (Horsley, Crane, Crabtree and Wood, 1983). Only if replicated findings are present across several studies under different as well as similar clinical conditions, can professionals be reassured that the information is credible and useful. Nursing researchers have historically conducted 'shotgun' research – one study in an area of interest followed by another study in another area of investigation. This pattern occurred for several reasons: first, that researchers were needed in a variety of roles – administrator, educator and clinician – and the research reflected changing interests and demands; secondly that researchers might only be able to conduct one or two studies and then have their energies diverted into other professional roles with an end to their research endeavours, and thirdly that nursing has not had a tradition of complete careers in science or building programmes of research due to scarce resources.

The lack of tradition and problem of scarce resources was well recognized by the professional leaders as hampering nursing development of its scientific base. The 1983 Institute of Medicine report on *Nursing and Nursing Education* in the United States included a recommendation to 'establish an organizational entity to place nursing research in the mainstream of scientific investigation.' An adequately funded focal point is needed at the national level to foster research that informs nursing and other health care practice and increases the potential for discovery and application of various means to improve patient outcomes. The National

Center for Nursing Research (NCNR) was established in order to provide a visible source of federal support for nursing research within the arena of biomedical and behavioural health care research and research training at the National Institutes of Health (NIH). Concurrently, a small but growing cadre of career nurse scientists was developing to conduct on-going research.

As resources and a cadre of career scientists are becoming available for nursing research, more programmes of research are evident. A programme of research includes a series of studies in a similar area of study, each of which builds on the prior investigation, both replicating and adding to the research question under study. An example of a programme of research is Johnson's series of studies investigating the relationship of sensory information to traumatic events (1987). The development of research programmes is crucial in terms of building depth in the science of nursing. As researchers develop each stage of their study based on the results of the last stage, information will be replicated, questioned and new areas of investigations will be explored.

As the cadre of career scientists increases within the nursing profession, depth in science will be accomplished through the researchers building on and replicating each others' studies. However, the breadth of nursing research is broad and 'natural' overlap in scientific areas may not occur rapidly enough to provide information needed for certain priority practice issues. Systematic targeting of specific priority areas for nursing practice and research will accelerate the development of depth in specified areas of high priority.

Depth in nursing science will also be facilitated by developing a body of information for nursing which is within the greater arena of other health care and basic science disciplines. The complex nature of nursing care issues and questions requires that knowledge from a number of biomedical behavioural sciences be understood and synthesized. Gortner (1980) and Hinshaw (1987) suggest that nursing is in a unique position to build and test knowledge which represents an interface of information from other disciplines and results in new understandings and essentially new knowledge generated from a nursing perspective. Due to the complexity of many care problems, access to the multiple health care and basic science disciplines is fundamental to the development of 'state of the art' nursing knowledge.

The challenge of being on the 'cutting edge' of knowledge development is facilitated by being in the mainstream of health care research. Nursing research cannot afford to be developed in a vacuum only to discover that valuable resources, such as time, energy and money have been spent in recreating information already known by other disciplines. In order to avoid this consequence, networks must be developed between scientists in similar areas of basic and applied study, across disciplines.

A tradition in nursing is developing which operationalizes the profession's commitment to excellence in the developing science of the discipline. The missions, programmes and initiatives of the National Center have been developed to facilitate and enhance the mandate to create and test a credible body of knowledge to guide nursing practice with an emphasis on improving care.

## NATIONAL CENTER FOR NURSING RESEARCH

The general purpose of the National Center for Nursing Research is the conduct and support of and dissemination of information respecting basic and clinical nursing research, training, and other programs in patient care research. A citation for this is Public Law 99–158. The goal of nursing research is to improve nursing care for all segments of society by expanding the scientific base for nursing practice. Nursing research recognizes the impact of biology and behaviour on health and recovery from illness. The rationale for placing a nursing research component in the National Institutes of Health was to incorporate nursing research into a broader-based, and more stable, funded health research environment. This move has made it possible for nursing science to continue its development in the context of other basic and clinical health research disciplines, and in surroundings that promote the scientific excellence of its growing body of knowledge. Nursing research, while building on the basic sciences, is concerned with health promotion, disease prevention, and the care and rehabilitation of patients. It compliments the NIH biomedical research orientation and as the scientific knowledge from a nursing perspective continues to develop and grow, it will be more accessible to those working in other disciplines as well as its own.

The mission of the National Institutes of Health is to provide leadership and direction to programmes designed to improve the health of the people of the United States through the following activities: (1) conducts and supports research into the causes, diagnoses, prevention and cure of diseases of man and the processes of human growth and development and the biological effects of environmental contaminates and in related sciences; and supports the training of research personnel, the construction of research facilities and the development of other research resources; (2) directs programmes for the collection, dissemination and exchange of information in medicine and health, including the development and support of medical libraries and the training of medical librarians and other health information specialists. Nursing research, like medical research, spans a wide range of investigative areas. Its focus is on developing knowledge about care of persons in health and disease in contrast to medical research, which emphasizes the diagnosis, prevention and treatment of disease. Care research is directed toward understanding the fundamental genetic, physiological, behavioural and environmental mechanisms that affect the ability of individuals, families and communities to maintain or enhance optimum functioning and minimize the negative effects of illness.

The National Center for Nursing Research has three major extramural programme areas: Health Promotion/Disease Prevention, Acute and Chronic Illness, and Nursing Systems. An extramural programme consists of awarding grants to nurse scientists in the academic and practice settings for research. The programme staff in the three content areas counsel nurses as they prepare and submit proposals requesting funds for support of research.

## Health promotion/disease prevention

The promotion of better health practices by individuals, families and communities is now recognized as a crucial public health objective. In recent years, there has been increased interest in self-care practices as alternative or supplemental choices to formal health care systems. The literature suggests that self-evaluation and treatment are the predominant forms of primary health care during periods of minor illness, and self-care is being used by a majority of the American population. Although there are fairly extensive data available on self-care as it relates to the taking of medications, very little is published about the range of self-care options in other areas. The need exists to identify and develop approaches for increasing individual and family awareness of the importance of personal habits and choices in maintaining good health. Because professional nurses, particularly public health nurses, are likely to have continuing front-line contact with the most vulnerable populations in terms of health, the National Center for Nursing Research supports research to increase the awareness of at-risk individuals about the power they have and the options available regarding their health.

The NCNR is interested in studies that identify health risk factors, design educational and intervention strategies to reduce health risks, and studies that determine the efficacy and cost-effectiveness of health promotion methodologies. Illustrative of the cost-effectiveness of such research is the finding of a project supported under this programme that identifies the beneficial effect of non-nutritive sucking on the digestion and weight gain of preterm infants which allows for earlier hospital discharge (Anderson, 1986). Researchers supported by the NCNR are studying the factors predictive of successful pregnancy and parenthood; analysing and developing interventions to help children and adolescents deal with the effects of stress, cope with chronic disability, and avoid inappropriate health related behaviours; and evaluating cultural beliefs about health and strategies for managing health problems in diverse ethnic groups. They are also developing nursing interventions for adults and the elderly in investigating their concepts of health, their health-related behaviours, and their use of health services.

## Acute and chronic illness

Nurses are studying the delivery and co-ordination of care to critically and chronically ill patients and their families. NCNR-supported investigators are examining the efficacy of structured educational programmes on managing the side effects of radiation therapy, and on patient outcomes following surgery and hospital discharge. Also being studied are the factors that predict which patients with chronic obstructive pulmonary disease will benefit the most from inspiratory muscle training. Health care problems of the ageing population being investigated are urinary incontinence, depression among nursing home residents, and the support and functioning of caregivers of elderly persons. Research on the care of children is also an important part of this programme, including studies of the care of children suffering from debilitating side effects of cancer, nursing procedures in neonatal intensive care units and the care of children with chronic illnesses. Other research is concerned with rehabilitation and cardiac disease, recovery following hip fracture, prevention and treatment of decubitus ulcers, the assessment of nursing procedures in acute illnesses such as endotracheal suctioning, the nasogastric and intestinal feeding tube placement, and the application of hypothermia blankets in patients with fever. The NCNR has joined other institutes at NIH in a programme announcement on pain and analgesia and is currently supporting research on the experience and treatment of pain.

## Nursing systems

The nursing systems area focuses on the structures and systems that facilitate the delivery of quality clinical care provided to patients in hospitals, nursing homes, other institutional settings and through home health and other community agencies. Without the appropriate elements in place, the effectiveness and quality of patient care can vary widely and perhaps unacceptably. The availability of nursing care and the quality of its delivery are recognized as important elements contributing to the patients' well-being. The preparation of family caregivers, the prevention of complications, and the efficient use of health resources are important areas of study. The examination of bioethical issues is also a component of the nursing systems programme. Advances in biomedical science, health care technology, and patient care delivery have contributed to the growing constellation of ethical issues that are confronting all health care providers. The appropriate level of technology, and the possible iatrogenic effects of technology, are high priority areas for nursing research.

Another critical area of research that cuts across all programme areas is concerned with acquired immune deficiency syndrome (AIDS). Estimates suggest that between 220 000 and 750 000 persons affected with HIV will require treatment in the United States between 1986 and 1991. A variety of studies have identified symptoms frequently experienced by HIV-infected individuals and AIDS patients, such as generalized lymphadenopathy, recurrent fevers, unintentional weight loss, diarrhoea, lethargy, skin lesions, respiratory distress and memory loss. There is little information available on the delivery of nursing care for patients with AIDS and their families, and on the techniques and procedures that are effective in the control of symptoms. Areas of research interests regarding AIDS include: skin care, nutritional measures to control weight loss, management of side effects of therapeutic agents, and interventions to address depression, anxiety, fear of death and other psychological symptoms. In particular, further research is needed to identify effective nursing approaches to achieving behavioural change in the various subgroups already infected or at risk for HIV infection. The NCNR has funded a study that follows HIV-positive infants and their mothers to address the infants' physical and developmental status and the mothers' physical and emotional status over time, and a project that will address patient care needs in different phases of HIV infection.

## Research support, research training and career development mechanisms

The NCNR offers several ways through which nurses and others can apply for support of nursing research projects. These mechanisms are the same used by other Institutes at NIH and vary by level of investigator's years since doctoral study.

*Research Project Grants (RO1).* These grants support discrete projects related to the investigator's interests and competence. The period of initial support may be up to five years.

*Academic Research Enhancement Award (AREA) (R15).* These grants support feasiblity studies and other small-scale research projects. Their purpose is to stimulate research of faculty members in educational institutions which historically have not been major participants in NIH programmes. Eligibility is limited to those domestic institutions that offer baccalaureate or advanced degrees in the sciences related to health, but have *not* received an NIH Biomedical Research Support Grant (BRSG) of $200 000 or more per year for four or more years during the period from fiscal year 1982 through fiscal year 1988. Awards may be up to $75 000 direct costs plus applicable indirect costs (not more than $35000 in any one year) for a period of up to three years. A single annual receipt date is designated for AREA applications.

*First Independent Research Support and Transition Award (FIRST) (R29).* These grants are intended to support the first independent investigative efforts of an individual and to help effect a transition toward the traditional types of NIH research project grants. FIRST awards are five-year awards. Total direct costs for the five-year period cannot exceed $350000. Principal Investigators must commit at least 50% of their time to the project in each budget period. When the proposed research project or programme is shorter than is appropriate for a FIRST award, new investigators are encouraged to consider using the traditional research project grant mechanisms.

*Programme Project Grant (P01).* These grants support a broadly based, often multidisciplinary, research programme with a specific major objective or theme. A programme project involves the organized efforts of groups of investigators who conduct discrete research projects related to the overall programme objective. The grant can provide support for the individual projects within the overall programme project, as well as for certain shared resources needed for the total research effort. Each individual project supported under a Programme Project Grant is expected to contribute to the overall programme objective.

*Co-operative Agreements (U01).* A co-operative agreement differs from a traditional research grant in that the NCNR staff participates in project planning and decision making to a greater extent than with a regular research grant. An investigator submits an application in response to a request for applications (RFA), issued by the NCNR or other NIH Institutes.

*Small Business Innovation Research Award (SBIR) (R43/R44).* These grants are made to small businesses that have the technological expertise to contribute to the research and development (R and D) mission of the NIH. Successful applications must involve research with the potential to lead ultimately to commercial products or services. Phase I supports the projects, limited in time and amount, to establish the technical merit and feasibility of R and D ideas. Phase II supports development of R and D ideas whose feasibility has been established in Phase I.

Nurses who are US citizens may also apply for funds to support their research training for both predoctoral and postdoctoral awards. In addition, awards are available to mid-career (career development) and senior scientist awards.

*Institutional National Research Service Award (NRSA) (T32).* Institutional training awards are made to eligible domestic institutions that have the required programme director, faculty, and facilities to provide relevant predoctoral and/or postdoctoral research training for nurses. Grant funds are primarily for trainee stipends, with a modest allowance to help defray necessary training-related costs.

The major distinction between the institutional and individual training awards is how the trainees are selected. In the case of institutional award, the award-receiving institution selects the trainees while in the case of an individual award (see below), the trainee is selected through direct application to the NIH.

*Individual NRSA Predoctoral Fellowship (F31).* These fellowship awards are available to support nurses for supervised research training, leading to a doctoral degree in areas related to the mission of the NCNR. Applicants must be registered nurses with either a baccalaureate degree in nursing and/or a master's degree in nursing.

*Individual NRSA Postdoctoral Fellowships (F32).* The postdoctoral fellowship is a priority of the NCNR. The purpose of these fellowship awards is to support the postdoctoral training (in areas related to the NCNR mission) of registered nurses holding a doctoral degree.

*Academic Investigator Award (AIA) (K07).* The Academic Investigator Award is a three-to-five-year award for junior faculty members, generally four to six years beyond the doctorate, who have demonstrated evidence of research potential. These awards are designed to allow promising nursing faculty members with research interest released time from administrative and teaching duties to establish their research programmes and mature into independent investigators. Support is provided to a maximum of $60 000 direct costs for salary, including applicable fringe benefits, as well as partial defrayment of research costs. Receivers of such an award commit at least 75% of their time to the conduct of a research project and related activities.

*Clinical Investigator Award (CIA) (K08).* The Clinical Investigator Award is designed to provide the opportunity for promising clinically-trained nurses to develop into independent investigators. Awards will be made to nurse investigators holding the doctorate to work under a sponsor at an NIH-supported Center programme or in one of the General Clinical Research Centers (GCRC) funded by the Division of Research Resources (DRR) of the National Institutes of Health. The provisions of the CIA are essentially the same as for the Academic Investigator Award.

*NRSA Senior Fellowship (F33).* These fellowship awards are designed to support nurse investigators who hold a doctoral degree and have generally had at least seven subsequent years of relevant research or professional experience at the time of the award. The award provides opportunities for experienced nurse scientists to make major changes in the direction of their research careers, to broaden their scientific background, to acquire new research capabilities, and to enlarge their command of an allied research field. It allows the recipient to take time from regular professional responsibilities to increase his/her capabilities for engaging in health-related research.

A number of awards are given for research support and training. Most of the research awards are single, investigator type (R01) with only a few programme projects or FIRST awards. There are a growing number of Small Business Innovation Research awards. In research training, most of the awards are for predoctoral education but there are a growing number of postdoctoral fellowships. A solid cadre of institutional awards have been allocated with further growth expected.

## INITIATIVES OF THE NCNR

Several initiatives have been outlined to guide the programmes of the NCNR and the allocation of resources to research support and training. These initiatives are focused on facilitating the nursing scientific community's response to the challenges involved in developing excellent science. The initiatives were developed to guide programmes which focus on building depth in nursing science and keeping research in the profession on the 'cutting edge' of knowledge frontiers. Five immediate and long-term initiatives have been identified: formation of the National Nursing Research Agenda, development of a career trajectory for research training, increased collaboration with other scientific disciplines, development of an intramural programme and development of an international programme.

The nursing scientific and professional community in the United States has been involved in the development of these initiatives. Since a major goal of the NCNR is facilitating a national research environment for nursing science, the profession's scientists were systematically included in the refinement and shaping of the NCNR initiatives and programmes.

## National Nursing Research Agenda

The National Nursing Research Agenda (NNRA) has several objectives; 'provide structure for selecting scientific opportunities and initiatives, promote depth in developing a knowledge base for nursing practice, and provide direction for nursing research within the discipline' (Hinshaw, Heinrich and Bloch, 1989). The major focus of the NNRA is the identification of the research priorities for the profession. This initiative is designed to develop depth in the knowledge base for nursing by allowing resources to be targeted to certain areas of research specified by the profession's educators, scientists and clinicians. By concentrating resources in several areas of research, scientists will be encouraged to conduct studies in a similar area of substantive content thus building a series of investigations from different and like perspectives. Over time, this targeting strategy will provide a depth of research in the specified areas from which accurate, reliable information can be transferred into practice.

The process for developing the NNRA has included several steps. First, a Steering Committee was formed from the NCNR staff and Advisory Council membership to plan and guide the formulation of the NNRA. Second, the broad research priorities were identified by a group of nurse scientists representing different clinical backgrounds and methodological expertise. Third, the Steering Committee members synthesized the broad priorities developed by colleagues with the priorities submitted by numerous professional organizations. From the synthesis process emerged several areas of priority for nursing research. The broad priority areas included:

*Low birth weight: mothers and infants.* This priority includes the study of the nursing care of prospective mothers at risk for having a low birth weight infant, with a focus on prevention of premature delivery; and of the care of low birth weight infants, with a focus on prevention of complications.

*HIV-positive patients, partners and families.* Prevention, ethical issues and physiological/psychosocial factors relating to care of persons with AIDS or HIV infection need to be examined.

*Long-term care for the elderly.* Possible areas of research to be developed include quality of nursing care, continuity of care, and iatrogenic complications. Important issues related to self-care, patient and caregiver coping and adaptation, and special populations such as the frail elderly need to be addressed.

*Symptom management.* The priority should blend biopsychosocial parameters of patient symptoms such as pain, fatigue, nausea and vomiting and include acute, chronic and terminal care. Measures for symptom assessment and management need to be developed.

*Information systems.* Standardized data sets which document nursing care across settings and a taxonomy to classify nursing phenomena and allow for the common use of terms is needed. The link(s) between resources and patient outcomes needs to be developed.

*Health promotion.* The critical issue for study is the psychosocial mechanisms underlying health promotion behaviours, with emphasis on lifestyle and the need to take responsibility for one's own health. Special population groups, such as children, need to be targeted.

*Technology dependency across the lifespan.* Interest is in technology dependency, individual and family responses to technology, and prevention of iatrogenic complications from the use of technology (Hinshaw, Heinrich and Bloch, 1989).

After the broad priorities were approved by the National Advisory Council for Nursing Research (NACNR), an expert panel was formed for each of the defined areas. The purpose of the panels is to evaluate and refine the broad priorities and recommend the areas for research in which nursing could make the most contribution in terms of the development of knowledge and the enhancement of practice. In addition, the expert panels are to evaluate and recommend the number and type of scientists needed to conduct the suggested research, and the resources needed for developing the research substantive area. This is the fourth step. Fifth, the recommendations from the expert panels will be formulated into programme announcements, using a variety of strategies, to stimulate research proposals in the recommended areas.

An updating mechanism will be part of the process formulating the NNRA. The initial research priorities are not all-encompassing but reflect only the top major areas of concern at this point in time. Practice issues will change and new areas of clinical concerns emerge, thus the formulation of new research priorities will be necessary.

It is important to note that only part of the NCNR resources will be focused on the defined priorities. While identifying priorities is important to building depth in the profession's knowledge base, it is also critical to be open to new and different areas of concern. Science is often best developed when the creative and innovative notions of the expert researcher are enhanced. Thus, resources also need to be available to facilitate such creative, innovative ideas for study.

## Career trajectory for research training and development

The second initiative is the formation of a career trajectory for research training and development. Essentially, the trajectory defines research training and career development as a continual part of a scientist's lifestyle. To remain on the 'cutting edge' of nursing science and research requires that an investigator have the newest, latest, state-of-the-art information in both the content and methodological aspects of their area of study. Remaining up-to-date in these areas requires continual attention to retraining with colleagues in nursing and in other disciplines.

The current major emphases in research training and career development are varied. One focus is on increasing the total cadre of predoctoral and postdoctoral fellows in order to increase the community of nurse scientists. An emphasis has been placed on increasing the number of post-doctorally-educated nurse scientists in order to facilitate new researchers' ability to start and sustain programmes of research (Stevenson, 1988). Such long-term programmes of research are basic to building depth in the body of knowledge. Opportunities also need to be available for colleagues of mid-career and senior level for their continual development in science. A number of strategies are offered to allow researchers in these stages of their career to obtain retraining or science opportunities working with other colleagues for achieving new knowledge and/or methodological skills. This emphasis enhances the nurse scientist's ability to stay on the 'cutting edge' of their research.

In addition, the National Research Service Award (NRSA) Institutional grants are emphasized since they provide research training within the context of an environment of scientific productivity with multiple faculty and a cadre of predoctoral and postdoctoral students. These awards are specific to research training in a particular substantive or methodological area, e.g., oncology, virology in relation to AIDS, and instrumentation or measurement of clinical phenomena.

## Collaboration for research

One of the principle purposes for the establishment of the National Center for Nursing Research within the National Institutes of Health was to place the profession's science development within the mainstream of the other health care scientific endeavours. The clinical questions with which professional nurses grapple, and thus the research questions which are raised and studied by the discipline's investigators are complex and multifaceted. The complexity requires that numerous perspectives reflecting both basic and applied sciences be brought to bear on the clinical issues which need to be studied.

Several collaborative endeavours have been initiated with other institutes at NIH. These include diverse projects such as nurse scientists working within the perinatal–neonatal centres of the National Institute of Child Health and Development, co-funding of a series of projects on urinary incontinence with the National Institute on Ageing, and co-sponsorship of several conferences with the National Institute of Allergy and Infectious Diseases to disseminate information to nurses and other health care providers about AIDS. Thus, collaboration has taken the form of co-funding extramural research projects, and co-sponsorship of conferences. A number of additional areas of study will be initiated to facilitate collaboration with the other institutes.

## Intramural research programme

An intramural research programme will be a major initiative for the National Center for Nursing Research within the next several years. This intramural programme would include basic and clinical research which could be actively conducted both at the Clinical Center, NIH, and with other health care agencies. An intramural research programme consists of scientists functioning as National Center for Nursing Research staff to conduct research within the clinical agencies or basic-science laboratories at the National Institutes of Health or collaborating institutions. Staff nurse researchers at the NCNR would investigate nursing care protocols which are of particular concern to the profession's mandate to society, related to a societal crisis in health care, and/or reflect an area of research not conducted by the discipline's extramural programme scientists.

Generally, the NIH intramural programmes have been based either within the laboratories of the individual institutes or are part of the intramural clinical research conducted at the Clinical Center. However, the National Center may wish to conduct its intramural programme within diverse health care settings, such as the home health care environment, skilled nursing homes, community hospitals, as well as public health care agencies, to name several. The NCNR intramural programme may actually reflect an organization 'without walls' concept which would facilitate investigations that could be conducted in different types of agencies, as well as promote research which studies the continuity and outcomes for clients as they are discharged from one level of care to another. In the interim, nurse scientists interested in working at the NIH Clinical Center or within existing institute intramural programmes are encouraged to work collaboratively with scientists in the other institutes at NIH. Several laboratories at NIH have identified interest areas and support for postdoctoral experiences for nurse scientists. The NCNR has issued a programme announcement to encourage nurse investigators to come to NIH to undertake studies in collaboration with other institutes.

## International programmes

With the discipline's emphasis on the cultural aspects of nursing care and the influence of such factors on practice, an international programme seems natural for the National Center for Nursing Research. Access to multiple populations from diverse cultures would allow the generation and testing of nursing science from many different perspectives. Interaction with colleagues from other countries would provide a rich context for the generation and dissemination of research issues.

The NCNR is working closely with the John F. Fogarty International Center at NIH. The Fogarty International Center for Advanced Study in the Health Sciences promotes international co-operation in the biomedical and behavioural sciences. This is accomplished primarily through long- and short-term fellowships and scientist exchanges.

Postdoctoral fellowship programmes are supported by the Fogarty International Center or by foreign governments and organizations. At a minimum, all provide stipend or *per diem* and international travel. Applications are reviewed for scientific merit by the Division of Research Grants, and funding decisions are made by the organizations that provide financial support. Opportunities for United States postdoctoral scientists include individual fellowship programmes and also senior international fellowship programmes. Nine countries support scientists who are US citizens or permanent residents to conduct collaborative research in laboratories in their countries. These include Finland, France, the Federal Republic of Germany, Ireland, Israel, Norway, Sweden, Switzerland, and Taiwan.

Opportunities for foreign postdoctoral scientists are also available through the Fogarty International Center. International research fellowships are awarded to provide opportunities for foreign scientists to extend their research experiences in US laboratories. Among other criteria, applicants to the programme must (1) be selected by the nominating committee in their country, (2) have ten years or less postdoctoral experience, (3) have a doctoral degree, (4) have demonstrated the ability to engage in independent basic or clinical research, (5) be invited by a scientist employed in a US non-profit institution, (6) have assurance from a non-profit institution in the home country of a position after completion of the fellowship, and (7) be proficient in spoken and written English. More than fifty countries/regions with nominating committees participate in this programme. The International Research Fellowship programme nominating committees were recently encouraged by the Fogarty International Center to make International Research Fellowships available to nurse scientists with doctoral degrees.

Bilateral exchange programmes are supported by the Fogarty International Center and co-operating foreign governments. The bilateral exchange programmes foster collaborative activities between well-qualified health professionals and biomedical students in the United States and participating countries in the study of health and biomedical problems that are of mutual interest and that lend themselves to a co-operative approach. Individuals from each country are supported for varying periods of work in the other country. Activities may include the sharing of consultative and technical advice that fosters individually conducted research in either country or joint research between collaborating scientists.

The National Institutes of Health also has on-going policies and procedures governing awards of research grants to foreign institutions and international organizations. 'For the purpose of advancing the status of health science in the United States (and thereby the health of the American people), the Secretary may participate with other countries in co-operative endeavours and biomedical research and the health services research and statistical activities' (NIH, 1983). In pursuing this objective, the NIH recognizes that it can support research in other countries only when such research has important specific relevance to the objectives of the NIH authorized in the legislation and appropriation acts of the Congress. Any exercise of this authority must be carried out in harmony with US foreign policy.

## CONCLUSION

Meeting the goal of 'Health for All' requires that the profession target major health concerns and develop innovative strategies for improving access to care and the quality of service. Developing innovative strategies will include the use of research to provide accurate reliable information relevant to the implementation of specific health care interventions. Providing research findings to guide practice involves facilitating the continuous study of the targeted health care priorities by the various disciplines. The major goal of the research programmes is to result in excellent scientific information which is ultimately transferable and relevant to health care practice.

## REFERENCES

Anderson, G. (1986) Pacifiers: the positive side. *Mat. Child Nurs.*, **11**, 122–4.
Cohen, B. (1984) Florence Nightingale. *Sci. Am.*, **250** (3), 1200–33.
Evans, J.R., Hall, K.L., and Warford, J. (1981) Shattuck Lecture – Health Care in the Developing World: Problems of Scarcity and Choice. *N. Engl. J. Med.*, **305**(19), 1117–27.
Gortner, S. (1980) Nursing science in transition. *Nurs. Res.*, **29**, 180–3.
Hinshaw, A.S. (1987, November) Integrating the Sciences and Humanities in Health Care. Presented as Annual Elizabeth Sterling Soule Lecture, University of Washington School of Nursing, Seattle.

Hinshaw, A.S., Heinrich, J., and Bloch, D. (1989) Evolving clinical nursing research priorities. *J. Profess. Nurs.*, **4**(6), 398, 458–9.

Horsley, J., Crane, J., Crabtree, K., and Wood, D.J. (1983) *Using Research to Improve Practice.* Grune & Stratton, Orlando, FL.

Institute of Medicine (1983) *Nursing and Nursing Education: Public Policies and Private Actions.* National Academy Press, Washington, DC.

Johnson, J.E. (1987) Effects of accurate expectations about sensations on the sensory and distress components of pain. *J. Pers. Soc. Psychol.*, **27**, 261–75.

National Institutes of Health (1983) Manual Transmittal 4104. National Institutes of Health, Bethesda, MD.

Stevenson, J.S. (1988) Nursing Knowledge Development: Into Era II. *J. Profess. Nurs.*, **4**(3), 152–62.

World Health Organization (1978) *Primary Health Care* (Report of the International Conference on Primary Health Care; Alma Ata, USSR), World Health Organization, Geneva.

World Health Organization (1986) *Regulatory Mechanisms for Nursing Training and Practice: Meeting Primary Health Care Needs.* World Health Organization, Geneva.

# CHAPTER FOUR

# Nursing research: cornerstone of nursing practice in Canada

*M. Josephine Flaherty*

There are many factors that have led to the belief of nurses and others that nursing research must be the cornerstone of nursing practice in Canada. The purpose of this chapter is to present a brief overview of the nursing research situation. The focus will be on events of last decade and their implications for nursing research in Canada as it is today. Comment will be made on the context of Canadian health care and nursing's place in it, needs and resources for nursing research, specific issues and events that have affected the development of nursing research in Canada, including the preparation of nurse researchers, and prospects for the future.

## The Canadian context of nursing

Nursing has a long and honoured history in Canada where the importance of health care and the role of nurses in it have been recognized since the early years of the seventeenth century when settlers from France, and later from other countries in Europe and the rest of the world, joined the indigenous peoples to form the basis for the multicultural Canada of today. Nursing in Canada began with the presence of religious Sisters from nursing orders and of Jeanne Mance, Canada's first lay nurse, among these first settlers from France. By the time of the English defeat of the French in the battle of the Plains of Abraham in 1759, the health care system in Canada was established firmly in a society that valued the health, well-being and religious life of its people and that transferred its concern for others into action. As a result, Canadian nursing, from its inception, attracted candidates of good character from reputable families and neither the status of nursing nor the level and quality of nursing service was subjected to the 'dark age' of nursing that was seen in the 'Sairy Gamp' era in Britain.

The need for health care services increased as settlers moved across

Canada and coped with hardships, poverty and serious sickness. Among the first pioneers in many parts of the country were nurses who were members of the congregation of The Grey Nuns of Montreal, the first non-cloistered order of Sisters to be founded, in 1738, in Canada. The Grey Nuns are seen as the first visiting nurses in the country; they provided nursing care to patients in their own homes in response to a need that was not being met by other nursing religious Sisters in Canada who were cloistered and who confined their activities to their hospitals. By the end of the nineteenth century, a new lay voluntary visiting nursing agency, the Victorian Order of Nurses (VON), that continues today to play a major role in Canadian community health nursing, was providing nursing care to people in various parts of the country, including, in 1898, to the pioneers who flocked to the northwestern outposts of Canada during the Klondike gold rush (Gibbon and Mathewson, 1947).

Today, in Canada, health is a provincial/territorial matter. Nurses are members of one of the five major health professions – and the largest one – in Canada. They are self-governing professionals who are responsible for the implementation of explicit and strong statutory provisions for the registration and regulation of members of the nursing profession in ten provinces and one territory (in the second territory, the Yukon, the first Nurses Act is before the territorial legislature awaiting approval). Under these statutes, Canadian nurses are recognized as independent and inter-dependent practitioners who are responsible and accountable for their own professional behaviour and who are expected to exercise the generally-accepted standards of nursing practice and to adhere to the codes of nursing ethics that have been identified by the nursing regulatory bodies. It should be noted that in all but four of the jurisdictions (British Columbia, Ontario, Manitoba and Saskatchewan), the legislation incorporates mandatory registration for nurses (Kerr, 1988a).

During the past twenty-five years, there have been significant changes in the roles of Canadian nurses and the nature and scope of nursing practice, including a trend towards specialization and credentialling. The Canadian Nurses Association (CNA) has been involved significantly in this (Kerr, 1988a; 1988c; Calkin, 1988).

## NURSING EDUCATION

As the need for nurses increased in the early years in Canada, it was recognized that a formal system of education for nurses was required. The influence of Florence Nightingale's work, particularly in English-speaking Canada, was seen in the founding of the first hospital-based diploma school of nursing in 1874 and of many other large and small schools during the next fifty years.

The quality of nursing education has been an on-going concern of the organized nursing profession in Canada. In the early part of the twentieth century, the need for improvement of nursing education was apparent and efforts were made to study the situation and to enhance the quality of the hospital-based nursing programmes.

The initiatives of the Canadian Nurses Association (CNA) and of the provincial nurses' associations have had significant impacts on the raising of educational standards in schools of nursing. For many years, there was discussion of the need for basic nursing education to be within the general education system and recommendations were made by individuals and groups in support of this. However, it was not until the sixties and seventies that most diploma nursing programmes in Canada were moved from hospitals to community college settings.

## HIGHER EDUCATION IN NURSING

Beginning in 1905 (MacMurchy, 1918; King, 1970), attempts were made by nursing associations to obtain advanced preparation for nurses. Years of effort resulted in approval in 1919 of the establishment of a Department of Nursing at the University of British Columbia and the first nursing degree programme was launched there soon afterward.

Following World War I, the Canadian Red Cross Society provided funds, for three years, for postgraduate instruction in public health nursing in five Canadian universities, Toronto, McGill, Alberta, Dalhousie and British Columbia (Gibbon and Mathewson, 1947). Departments of nursing were formed in these and several other Canadian universities within the next few years (Gibbons and Mathewson, 1947).

It was demonstrated at the University of Toronto, beginning in the mid-twenties, that nurses could be prepared in an effective and educationally sound manner in a university school with the university directing and controlling all the courses in the programme. The Report of the Royal Commission on Health Services (1964) recommended that ten more university nursing programmes be established, that non-integrated programmes be eliminated as soon as possible and that baccalaureate programmes be expanded to enable them to prepare approximately one-fourth of the basic nursing students in Canada (1964, vol. 1). Within a few years, new university schools were established and most basic programmes became integrated (Kerr, 1988d).

## EDUCATIONAL STATUS OF NURSES IN CANADA

In 1988, 210923 nurses were employed in Canada to meet the needs of a population of 26565375, thus providing a ratio of 1 nurse to 125 population; the ratio was 1:142 in 1982.

In 1970, 7% of nurses employed in nursing in Canada had baccalaureate or higher degrees; this figure had risen to 10% by 1980 and to 13% in 1986 (Statistics Canada, 1988). By 1987, approximately 14% (26 177) of nurses employed in nursing had educational preparation at the baccalaureate or higher levels. Of these, over one-half (54.1%) reported that they were in general duty/staff nurse positions, providing direct patient care in hospitals, nursing homes/homes for the aged and in the community. Almost 12% were employed in nursing education and almost 20% were in administrative positions ranging from head nurses to directors of nursing.

Seventy per cent of these nurses were employed in hospitals, 2% were in nursing homes/homes for the aged and 24.4% were in community health (Canadian Nursing Association, 1988a).

In 1986, the number of nurses employed in Canada prepared at the master's or higher levels was 1853 (less than 0.9%) (Statistics Canada, 1988).

In 1986, the last year for which statistics on doctoral level preparation of nurses in Canada are available, the number of nurses with earned doctorates, who were living and working in Canada, was 193, in contrast to 124 in 1982 and 81 in 1980. The net increase between 1980 and 1982 was 53% while the increase between 1982 and 1986 was 56% (Stinson, MacPhail and Larsen, 1988).

In 1980, 70% of doctorally prepared nurses in Canada were employed in nursing positions; the comparable figures for 1982 and 1986 were 74% and 80%. The latter figure includes five nurses who were self-employed in nursing positions. Details about the types of employment, geographical locations, types and disciplines of the doctoral degrees, ages, countries in which degrees were obtained and language facility of the doctorate holders are provided by Stinson, MacPhail and Larsen (1988). It is interesting to note that over half (n=110) of the doctoral degrees were obtained in a 7-year period (1980–1986) and 44% (n=84) were obtained in a twenty-year period preceding that (1960–1979) (Stinson, MacPhail and Larsen, 1988).

By 1988, there were 27 university schools of nursing in Canada, of which 21 offered basic (generic) baccalaureate programmes, 25 offered post-RN baccalaureate programmes and 11 offered Master's programmes in nursing; one university (McGill) had two 'special case' students enrolled in a doctoral programme in nursing (Canadian Association of University Schools of Nursing, 1988). McMaster University offered a master's degree in health sciences with a major focus in nursing.

It should be noted that in 1982, 6621 students graduated from diploma schools of nursing in Canada; these numbers remained fairly stable over the next five years and in 1986, there were 6762 graduates (Statistics Canada, 1988).

In 1982, there were 1023 graduates of basic baccalaureate programmes in nursing; these numbers rose slowly to only 1249 in 1986 (Statistics Canada, 1988).

At the end of 1987, there were 9606 students enrolled in baccalaureate programmes in nursing in Canada; 5351 were in basic (generic) programmes and 4255 were in post-RN baccalaureate programmes. At the end of 1987, there were 729 students enrolled in master's programmes in nursing in Canada and two 'special case' students in a doctoral programme (Canadian Association of University Schools of Nursing, 1988).

In 1982, there were 2316 full-time teachers in diploma schools of nursing. Of these, 7 had doctoral degrees, 295 had master's preparation, 1523 had baccalaureates and 491 had no degrees. The comparable figures for 1986 were: total 416; doctorate 0; master's 38; baccalaureate 250; no degree 119; unknown 9.

In 1982, in the university programmes, there were 584 teachers, of whom 67 held doctoral degrees, 393 master's degrees, 123 baccalaureates and 1 had no degree. In 1986, the comparable figures were: total 613; doctorate 115; master's 424; baccalaureate 65; no degree 0; unknown 9 (Statistics Canada, 1988).

The supply of nurses graduated from or studying in doctoral and master programmes, represents a considerable potential for nursing research.

## EDUCATION FOR ENTRY TO NURSING PRACTICE

In both the United States and Canada, there has been discussion for some time of the raising of the educational requirements for entry to nursing practice to the baccalaureate level. In Canada, this position on entry to practice began in 1932 with the Weir Report, *Survey of Nursing Education in Canada* which recommended that schools of nursing be incorporated in the general education system and be subsidized by government funds (Canadian Nurses Association 1968). The decisions of the Alberta Association of Registered Nurses in 1975 and of the Canadian Nurses Association in 1982 to endorse the baccalaureate standard began what has been termed 'the most contentious issue in the history of nursing in this country' (Besharah, 1981).

A background paper published by the CNA in 1982 gives the historical perspective and a clear rationale for the Association's position (Canadian Nurses Association, 1982). Updates of the situation are provided bi-monthly in the *Entry to Practice Newsletter* (Canadian Nurses Association, 1985a to present).

Most provincial nurses' associations have endorsed the CNA's stand, but the discussion continues, with both sides of the question being debated by nurses, provincial governments and other individuals and groups. Whether or not the baccalaureate standard will be realized by the year 2000 remains to be seen but it is believed that there is growing support for the position. The issue has been discussed and documented by a number of authors such as Kerr (1988d) and Rovers and Bajnok (1988) and in several series of bulletins from the CNA and from provincial and territorial nurses associations.

## NURSING RESEARCH

Although Canadian nurses have been involved in research for more than half a century, in the beginning their research activity consisted largely of co-operation with and/or assistance to members of other disciplines. The Weir Report (1932), referred to above, was a major study of nursing education in Canada conducted by a non-nurse investigator who was engaged jointly by the Canadian Nurses Association (CNA) and the Canadian Medical Association (CMA). For some years, even after the first master's programme in nursing in Canada was founded in 1959, most nursing studies were related to nursing education, nursing administration or public health, the functional areas that were the focus of graduate education in nursing. With the opening of more master's programmes in nursing, however, interest in the study of clinical practice issues grew and nursing research was directed increasingly to nursing practice issues (Griffin, 1971; Imai, 1971). By the 1970s, the majority of nursing research studies in Canada were in this area (Stinson, 1986).

Growth of nursing research activity in Canada has been gradual, in pace with the slow increase in the size of the pool of qualified nurse researchers. Much of the research takes place in university settings where graduate programmes are located and many nurses with higher levels of education are found. A major challenge is the preparation of nurse researchers and the Canadian Nurses Association has played a major role in the promotion of this and other dimensions of the development of nursing research.

## Activities of the Canadian Nurses Association in nursing research

Although the Canadian Nurses Association has declared that 'Research in nursing is needed to improve the quality of nursing care and to contribute to the efficiency and effectiveness of health care and the quality of life of Canadians' (Canadian Nurses Association, 1985b), many nurses in Canada do not regard research as necessary to their practice. In light of this, for some years, the CNA has focused attention on nursing research and has worked actively with other organizations towards the development of a 'nursing research reality', that is, 'the establishment of a general expectation among nurses, governments and the public of nursing research as a basic core of the discipline, for example, the institutionalization or imperative for research' (Canadian Nurses Organization, 1984). A number of issues in nursing research in Canada were identified over several decades and action was taken on them by various groups and with varying degrees of success in achievement of the objectives. Some of these issues and activities will be identified here, together with brief discussion of the objectives and strategies that were developed and implemented in relation to them.

## THE CNA LIBRARY

Until 1969, CNA's involvement in nursing research focused on the development of the CNA Library as the most outstanding collection of nursing literature in Canada (MacPhail, 1988a). In 1969, the CNA stated to the Special Senate Committee on Science Policy that research in nursing practice and more prepared nurse researchers were essential to the provision of health care for Canadians (Canadian Nurses Association, 1981).

## THE CANADIAN NURSES FOUNDATION

In 1962, the Canadian Nurses Foundation (CNF) was established to provide financial support for education of nurses at baccalaureate and higher levels; the Foundation began to provide small nursing research project grants in 1982. The CNA provided the sum of $10000 in support of the CNF (MacPhail, 1988a).

## NATIONAL NURSING RESEARCH CONFERENCES

Between 1971 and 1987, ten national nursing research conferences were held in Canada, each one sponsored by a host university on a volunteer basis, and CNA has supported these strongly (MacPhail, 1988a, 1988c). These conferences were supported financially, in varying amounts and patterns, by the Department of National Health and Welfare, by provincial nurses' associations and governments and by registration fees of participants (MacPhail, 1988c). The proceedings of nine of these conferences have been published. The CNA has published research abstracts and a few research articles in *The Canadian Nurse* Journal.

## CNA COMMITTEE ON NURSING RESEARCH

In 1971, CNA established a Special Committee on Nursing Research, which later became a standing committee, to assist the Board in the development and implementation of research policy and to advise the Board on research matters. In 1976, a Member-at-large for Nursing Research was added to the CNA Board of Directors.

The Standing Committee on Nursing Research has been working on the development, implementation and on-going updating of the 'Research Imperative for Nursing in Canada: A 5-Year Plan Towards the Year 2000' (Canadian Nurses Association, 1984), the overall aim of which is to achieve a scientific foundation for nursing practice.

Specific terms of reference for the CNA Standing Committee on Nursing Research may be set for each biennium. For the 1988–1990 biennium they are to: (1) provide consultation and advice to the Board of Directors and staff in relation to research and research matters, and (2) examine the Research Imperative for Nursing and make recommendations for follow-up, with particular consideration of: (a) funding and nursing participation in funding agency decision making, (b) a nursing research reality including strategies to facilitate research utilization on clinical settings, and (c) the structure within CNA for the continuing advance of research in nursing.

The CNA Research Imperative has three major goals with several objectives within each goal. These goals and objectives will be presented and comments made on activities and results related to each.

## Goal I. To develop Nurse Researchers

To accomplish this the Research Imperative proposes three objectives:

*(1) The establishment of nursing doctoral programmes in Canadian universities.* The CNA hoped to see the development of a blueprint for systematic establishment of doctoral programmes and has communicated with the Canadian Association of University Schools of Nursing (CAUSN) regarding this. CNA has encouraged university schools of nursing in their efforts to establish doctoral programmes in nursing. In 1978, the CNA sponsored a National Seminar on Doctoral Preparation for Canadian Nurses and published the Proceedings (Zilm, Larose and Stinson, 1979). Following this seminar, CNA, CNF and CAUSN developed a proposal, 'Operation Bootstrap', and sought $5.2 million from the W.K. Kellogg Foundation for establishment grants for PhD in Nursing programmes, two nursing research consortia, emergency fellowships for doctoral preparation as well as funding for communicating nursing research and for maintaining an inventory of nurses with doctoral preparation. The funds were not obtained from the Kellogg Foundation and by the end of 1988, a doctoral programme in nursing had not been established in Canada (MacPhail, 1988a).

In 1980, the University of Montreal and McGill University proposed a joint, bilingual doctoral programme in nursing which was not approved at the time; work is continuing in both universities towards the establishment of PhD in Nursing programmes and it is believed that support is growing for them. Two 'special case' nursing students are enrolled at McGill in PhD programmes. A 1980 proposal at the University of Toronto did not receive full approval but selected nurses have been studying toward and completing doctoral programmes there, in the Institute of Medical Science, in subject areas that are related closely to nursing.

In 1986, a proposed PhD in Nursing programme was approved by the Board of Governors at the University of Alberta but by autumn 1989, the Alberta government had not provided funds to implement it. (MacPhail, 1988a, Stinson, Field and Thibaudeau, 1988). The CNA continues to lobby strongly for doctoral education in nursing in Canada by encouraging universities to establish programmes, requesting funding agencies to provide funds and sensitizing governments and provincial/territorial nurses' organizations to the needs and resources for this level of education. At conferences, workshops and symposia, the CNA proposes strategies for optimum use of existing human, physical and fiscal resources such as joint appointments, consortium approaches and satellite mechanisms to permit wide exposure for students to different philosophies of science and researchers.

*(2) The establishment of post-doctoral programmes in nursing in Canadian universities.* The CNA had hoped to see in place in the eighties opportunities for post-doctoral studies that would forge nursing research, practice, theory links and/or interdisciplinary research and CNA continues to encourage establishment of such arrangements. In order to inform nurses about financial resources, the CNA published a 'Sources of Funds' document in 1984 and updates it biannually (Canadian Nurses Association, 1988b). To encourage the availability of assistance to prospective recipients of financial assistance, the CNA has been sending information to Deans/Directors of schools of nursing to promote successful applications for scholarships.

A major effort of the CNA has been its lobbying for increased funding for studentships and research awards for nurses; the Medical Research Council (MRC), the major granting agency for medical research, has been the target of major attention. This resulted in 1988 in changes in the eligibility criteria for MRC studentships to allow applications from nurses holding an MSc or equivalent. The National Health Research and Development Programme (NHRDP), which has been the major source of funding for nursing research awards, and the MRC announced in 1988 a special joint development programme to promote nursing research. Funds may be requested by Deans responsible for schools of nursing for: (1) salary support for independent investigators who devote at least 75% of their time to research and who secure funds for support of their research; (2) operating funds for up to three years; support for continuation after three years of such research may be sought through the regular programmes of MRC or NHRDP; and (3) the costs of equipment required for the research to be undertaken (Canadian Nurses Association, 1988c, unpublished typescript).

To promote a variety of opportunities to post-doctoral research training for nurses, the CNA is in the process of establishing a database of experienced nurse researchers and theorists with whom candidates could study and it is hoped that this will be completed early in 1989.

*(3) Creation of career development opportunities for nurse researchers.* With a view to increasing the proportion of nurses holding 'career awards' and to achieving increased funding for established on-going career awards, CNA lobbied successfully for changes in the MRC grants and awards guide that remove the previous barriers to nurses' applications. To encourage the likelihood of nurses receiving research funding, experienced nurse researchers are encouraging present and potential nurse researchers to apply for research awards and are assisting them in the development of proposals and applications for funding.

## Goal II. Development of Nursing Research

Four objectives are specified towards achievement of this goal:

*(1) Establishment of stable adequate nursing research funding at all levels with a suggested pool of $12 million by 1989.* To this end, the CNA has worked successfully for the appointment of a nurse to the Council of the MRC to ensure that the presence of nursing as a research discipline is perceived by the Council and to advocate for funding for worthy nursing research projects. The CNA submits briefs to appropriate bodies and initiates and participates in discussions of nursing research needs and resources with government and other funding officials and groups. In investigating annual federal/provincial funding earmarked and awarded for nursing research, the CNA has discovered that these amounts have increased from $659 597 in 1980–81 to $1 101 016 in 1987–1988 (unpublished data).

The CNF established 'small research grants awards' in 1984 and had awarded a total of $27 836 to the end of 1988. Since additional funds have been obtained in a recent corporate fundraising appeal, the Foundation will be able to increase its level of funding. The Association is encouraging universities, health care agencies and other organizations, such as major foundations and corporations, to make trust funds for research accessible to nursing and some progress is being made. To increase public awareness of nursing research, information and interpretive brochures have been developed and circulated by the CNA (Canadian Nurses Association, 1988b).

Funding for nursing research has not been earmarked for nursing research at provincial levels with one exception – the Alberta Government's commitment of one million dollars to nursing research during 1982–1987 (Stinson, Field and Thibaudeau, 1988). Its later decision to continue to fund the Alberta Foundation for Nursing Research (AFNR) grants programme has resulted in the 1988 awards taking the AFNR funding for nursing research over the one million dollar mark since the Foundation was established in 1982 (Alberta Foundation for Nursing Research, 1988).

*(2) Increase of access of nurses to sources of funding.* The CNA's nomination of nurse researchers to federal funding councils has resulted in three nurses being appointed to MRC review committees. Similar appointments have been made to provincial research funding review boards and other funding organization boards through the efforts of CNA member associations and other groups. In 1987, the CNA sponsored a Research Consultation to assist nurse investigators develop skills and project proposals, with the result that collaborative projects were developed.

*(3) Increase of the number and quality of projects and nursing research programmes.* There has been encouragement of nursing research development grants to universities and agencies and promotion of co-operation and collaboration among workers and institutions. Research institutes have been established in affiliation with several universities and at least one more is in the process of development. There has been discussion of the feasibility of establishment of a Canadian centre for research in nursing and/or of nursing research consortia.

To encourage applications for research funding and training, information about sources of funds has been gathered and circulated biannually since 1984. To increase knowledge about and the quality of nursing research projects, the CNF held a 'Reunion of Scholars' in 1987, with financial support from NHRDP, MRC and the Secretary of State. Twelve CNF scholars presented nursing papers that were discussed by a very active group of nurse researcher participants.

*(4) Provision of leadership in the pursuit of excellence in nursing research and scholarship.* The CNA, in co-operation with other groups, is encouraging the sharing of expertise by nurse researchers and scholars and the identification and increase of the visibility and accessibility of nursing research role models. Reference has been made to the compilation of data about doctorally prepared nurses (Stinson, MacPhail and Larsen, 1988). A Canadian Nursing Research Group has been formed that meets periodically and communicates through a newsletter.

## Goal III: To develop a nursing research reality

The Research Imperative identifies five objectives towards the meeting of this goal:

*( 1 )  The establishment within the CNA of ways and means to co-ordinate and implement the goals of the Research Imperative.* A research officer position provides personnel to manage the research effort, to work closely with the CNA Research Committee and to keep abreast of and exchange information about research policies and activities of national and provincial/territorial nursing organizations.

*( 2 )  Establish structures for the conduct of nursing research in institutions.* Efforts have been made to increase the number of nursing research positions in institutions through increasing the level of awareness in agencies of the need for and roles of persons filling these positions and identification of strategies for optimum use of resources. Nurses are encouraged to use opportunities to communicate information about nursing research roles through the literature and through large and small conferences and workshops and to promote the development and implementation of nursing research policies in all nursing practice and education venues. More nursing research positions are being established and nurses are more inclined than they were in the past to ask researchable questions and to take part in nursing investigations.

*( 3 )  Promote development of a research focus in educational programmes.* On-going efforts are being made to raise the level of awareness of nurses of the educational preparation required for nursing research and the usefulness of and relevance of nursing research for nursing practice. A pamphlet on nursing research was prepared by the CNA and circulated in CNA journals. A research orientation is encouraged for all baccalaureate and master's programmes with a view to promotion of understanding by all nurses of nursing research and its place in nursing. Schools of nursing are urged to include students in research activities, to support student research efforts and to conduct seminars and discussion groups for staff and students about on-going and completed nursing research.

*( 4 )  Improve communication of nursing research activities and findings.* Nurse researchers are encouraged to deposit copies of research reports in the CNA Library and an Index of Canadian Nursing Studies is prepared annually by CNA Library staff. A refereed research edition of *The Canadian Nurse* journal was published in 1984.

Although *Nursing Papers*, a journal devoted to nursing research, has been in existence for some years, it was not until 1986 that it was sub-titled *The Canadian Journal of Nursing Research* to convey clearly its nature and purpose. To date, its circulation is under 1000 and this must be increased substantially if the journal is to remain viable and to serve its purpose of disseminating information about nursing research. It should be noted that in 1987, the cost of a subscription to this journal was half of the cost of a subscription to *Nursing Research* and one-fifth of that of *Research in Nursing and Health*, both of which are published in the United States (MacPhail, 1988b).

*(5) Create and promote the image of a research orientation in nursing to nurses, to other disciplines and to the public.* A plan to market widely the notion, the need and the utility of higher education, research and scholarly activity in nursing must be developed and implemented in Canada. Individuals and groups are being encouraged to work in co-operation with the CNA's communication structures, to collaborate with print, radio and television media and to make nursing scientific activities and nurse scientists visible and accessible to the public.

## PROSPECTS FOR THE FUTURE

Although a great deal of progress has been made in nursing research in Canada during the past couple of decades in general (Kerr, 1986; Stinson, 1986; Ritchie, 1988; MacPhail, 1988c), Canadian nursing research has a long way to go. The establishment of the scientific base for nursing practice is not moving quickly enough (Ritchie, 1988). Young and not so young nurses must be groomed at all levels to see the relevance of nursing research for the enhancement of their practice and to consider seriously becoming involved in research activities. Efforts must be made to promote the application of research findings in day-to-day practice (MacPhail, 1988b) and competent nurse researchers must be prepared and given opportunities to engage in meaningful research. The state of research funding for nursing must be examined (Kerr, 1986; 1988b) and steps taken to bring it to appropriate levels. Efforts must be made to document the extent of nursing research in Canadian hospitals (Thurston, Tenove and Church, 1987) and other institutions and to increase the activity in it.

Nursing research is every nurse's business in Canada and members of the profession must be helped to see and appreciate this and to help the researchers to ensure that the problems being investigated are relevant ones and that the findings are put to use. Until all Canadian nurses accept this challenge and commit themselves to the task, the scientific foundation of nursing will not become the cornerstone of nursing practice in Canada.

## REFERENCES

Alberta Foundation for Nursing Research (1988) AFNR funding reaches $1 million. Press release, July 19, 1988, Edmonton, Alberta.

Besharah, A. (1981) When will the shouting start? *Can. Nurse*, **77**(3), 6.

Calkin, Joy D. (1988) Specialization in nursing practice, in *Canadian Nursing Faces the Future* (eds J. Baumgart and J. Larsen), C.V. Mosby, Scarborough, Ont. pp. 279–295.

Canadian Association of University Schools of Nursing (CAUSN) (1988) Statistics on university enrolments and faculty, unpublished data.

Canadian Nurses Association (1968) The leaf and the lamp. Ottawa.

Canadian Nurses Association (1981) The seventh decade 1969–1980, Ottawa.

Canadian Nurses Association (1982) Entry to the practice of nursing: A background paper, Ottawa.

Canadian Nurses Association (1984) The research imperative, Ottawa.

Canadian Nurses Association (1985a to present) Entry to practice newsletter, vol. 4, no. 2, April, 1988, Ottawa.

Canadian Nurses Association (1985b) A statement on research in nursing, Ottawa, Author.

Canadian Nurses Association (1988a) Entry to practice newsletter, vol. 4, no. 3, June, 1988, Ottawa.

Canadian Nurses Association (1988b) Sources of funds for nursing education and nursing and health-related research projects, Ottawa.

Canadian Nurses Association (1988c) NHRDP – MRC joint programme: development of research on nursing. Typescript. Ottawa.

Gibbon, J.M. and Mathewson, M.S. (1947) *Three Centuries of Canadian Nursing*, MacMillan, Toronto.

Griffin, A. (1971) Nursing research in Canadian universities, in *First National Conference on Research in Nursing Practice*, University of British Columbia, pp. 94–122. School of Nursing, Vancouver.

Imai, H.R. (1971) Professional associations and research activities in nursing in Canada, in *First National Conference on Research in Nursing Practice* University of British Columbia School of Nursing, Vancouver, pp. 89–93.

Kerr, J.C. (1986) Structure and funding of nursing research in Canada, in *International Issues in Nursing Research* (eds S.M. Stinson and J.C. Kerr), Croom Helm, London, pp. 97–112.

Kerr, J.C. (1988a) Professionalization in Canadian nursing, in *Canadian Nursing Issues and Perspectives* (eds. J. Kerr and M. MacPhail), McGraw-Hill Ryerson, Toronto, pp. 27–34.

Kerr, J.C. (1988b) The financing of nursing research in Canada, in *Canadian Nursing Issues and Perspectives* (eds J. Kerr and M. MacPhail), McGraw-Hill Ryerson, Toronto, pp. 113–122.

Kerr, J.C. (1988c) Credentialing in nursing, in *Canadian Nursing Issues and Perspectives* (eds J. Kerr and M. MacPhail), McGraw-Hill Ryerson, Toronto, pp. 309–318.

Kerr, J.C. (1988d) Entry to practice: striving for the baccalaureate standard, in *Canadian Nursing Issues and Perspectives* (eds J. Kerr and M. MacPhail), McGraw-Hill Ryerson, Toronto, pp. 259–266.

Kerr, J.C. (1988e) The growth of graduate education in nursing in Canada, in *Canadian Nursing Issues and Perspectives* (eds J. Kerr and M. MacPhail), McGraw-Hill Ryerson, Toronto, pp. 353–372.

King, M.K. (1970) The development of university nursing education, in M.Q. Innis (ed), *Nursing Education in a Changing Society* (ed. M.Q. Innis) University of Toronto Press, Toronto, pp. 67–85.

MacMurchy, H. (1918) University training for the nursing profession. *Can. Nurse,* **14**(9), 1284–1285.

MacPhail, J. (1988a) The role of the Canadian Nurses Association in the development of nursing in Canada, in *Canadian Nursing Issues and Perspectives,* (eds J. Kerr and M. MacPhail), McGraw-Hill Ryerson, Toronto, pp. 35–46.

MacPhail, J. (1988b) Research-mindedness in the profession, in *Canadian Nursing Issues and Perspectives* (eds. J. Kerr and M. MacPhail), McGraw-Hill Ryerson, Toronto, pp. 99–112.

MacPhail, J. (1988c) Scope of research in nursing practice, in *Canadian Nursing Issues and Perspectives,* (eds J. Kerr and M. MacPhail), McGraw-Hill Ryerson, Toronto, pp. 123–133.

Ritchie, J.A. (1988) Research and nursing practice, in *Canadian Nursing Faces the Future* (eds A.J. Baumgart and J. Larsen), C.V. Mosby, Scarborough, Ont., pp. 245–261.

Rovers, Ria and Bajnok, Irmajean (1988) Educational preparation for entry into the practice of nursing, in *Canadian Nursing Faces the Future* (eds A.J. Baumgart and J. Larsen), C.V. Mosby, Toronto, pp. 323–335.

*Royal Commission on Health Services Vol. I* (1964) Queen's Printer, Ottawa.

Statistics Canada (1988) *Nursing in Canada 1986,* Ottawa, Author.

Stinson, S.M. (1986) Nursing research in Canada, in *International Issues in Nursing Research* (eds M.S. Stinson and J.C. Kerr), pp. 236–258.

Stinson, S.M., Field, P.A. and Thibaudeau, M.-F. (1988) Graduate education in nursing, in *Canadian Nursing Faces the Future* (eds A.J. Baumgart and J. Larsen) C.V. Mosby, Toronto, pp. 337–361.

Stinson, S.M., MacPhail, J. and Larsen, J. (1988) *Canadian Nursing Doctoral Statistics: 1986 Update,* Canadian Nurses Association, Ottawa.

Thurston, N.E., Tenove, S. and Church, J. (1987) Nursing research in Canadian teaching hospitals. Department of Nursing, Foothills Provincial General Hospital and Faculty of Nursing, University of Calgary, Calgary, Alberta.

Weir, G. (1932) *Survey of Nursing Education in Canada,* University of Toronto Press, Toronto.

Zilm, G., Larose, O. and Stinson, S. (1979) *PhD (Nursing),* Canadian Nurses Association, Ottawa.

# CHAPTER FIVE

# Nursing research in Jamaica: catalyst and partner in health policy

*Syringa Marshall Burnett*

'We must recognize that a profession is committed to the task of enlarging the body of knowledge it applies to the problems and troubles with which it deals' – Robert Merton – (Address to the 41st Convention of the American Nurses Association (ANA) June 1958).

Over the past four decades nurses have correctly displayed increasing interest in the development of a body of knowledge and legitimizing the right to academic and professional status through research.

In the postwar period tremendous scientific and technological achievements have literally forced nurses to take notice and respond. The fact that other disciplines were not only making phenomenal progress but achieving considerable credibility, status and recognition through research, was not entirely lost on nurses though slowly absorbed initially. As the research successes of other disciplines began to influence nursing and the benefits were perceived, the realization of the potential inherent in the use of the scientific method grew. A whole new generation of research-minded nurses was bred.

In every country nurses are attempting to master the scientific method. Though the pace varies, nurses universally are much more research oriented now than previously. Today there are unmistakable signs that nurses are achieving research competence, eloquence, literacy and leadership. The issue is no longer the justification for nurses doing research and building a corpus of nursing science. The current concern is the utilization of findings that are relevant, appropriate, valid and reliable to guide practice, influence policy and direct change.

There is general consensus that whereas only some nurses may choose to be researchers, all nurses should be good consumers of research. The teaching of research invariably addresses this objective and the differences in the knowledge base necessary for consumption as distinct from investigation are made clear.

But to what purpose do we consume? Is it for knowledge and insight alone? Or can it be that beyond our understanding of the research report (written or oral) and our ability to critically evaluate its quality there may perchance be a responsibility to act on what we now know.

There is for example concern expressed regarding the lack of adequate replication of research, no doubt influenced by such criteria as 'original' work for theses and dissertations. But external to academia, do consumers have a role to test findings? What if having carefully read about the indicators for potential decubiti and the preventive role of timed repositioning, nurse consumers were to begin testing this in their own environment? Such findings would certainly have the potential for application where people prone to decubiti are under the care of nurses.

Another fruitful area that has general acceptance is the now recognized positive relationship between preoperative preparation and the postoperative outcomes for patients. Not only do nursing schools teach this but the nursing care actions of different groups such as operating theatre nurses and nurse anaesthetists (as well as ward and clinic staff) include this important practice.

As the leaders in nursing research extend their horizons and document their findings the ripple effect is extending universally. Nurses are exercising increasing vigour in nursing research.

## DEVELOPMENT OF NURSING RESEARCH

The development of nursing research in Jamaica (and the Caribbean) has similarities to the experience of nurses elsewhere. Very little was said or written and even less done about the subject until fairly recently. Nursing research remains in its infancy even in 1989, lagging behind the successes recorded by many other countries.

As a British colonial outpost, the influence and impact of Florence Nightingale was ever present but primarily manifested in the rigid authoritarian style of nursing service and training. Nurses were socialized to an understanding of Florence Nightingale as 'the lady with the lamp' who had great concern for patients, willingly worked long and inconvenient hours, did not expect even basic necessities, was unconcerned with material benefits and used simple effective measures to improve the environment. These characteristics summarized by the word 'dedication' projected a powerful image which was to influence all aspects of nursing for generations. Nurses did as they were told and did not ask questions. Even when Florence Nightingale's philosophy and practice were revisited, the emphasis was on education.

It has therefore been for many nurses a real shock, albeit quite inspirational, to learn that Florence Nightingale was also an assertive, clear-thinking, brilliant, well-educated woman of independent means, who conducted research, made statistical analyses and used her new knowledge as irrefutable evidence to influence public policy and change; that she understood the bureaucracy and the political powers of her day and exploited these for reform in health care. Furthermore, she wrote extensively, leaving substantial primary sources of information.

If there was only a partial view of Florence Nightingale's contribution which obscured her research capabilities and the use to which she put her findings, then it is not difficult to understand the drought of information on our own Mary Seacole. It is the nature of colonization that history is written from the colonizers point of view (Columbus 'discovered' Jamaica and all that)! Today we realize that Mary Seacole was well known and respected in many Caribbean countries and Central America prior to her sojourn in the Crimea (where she met Florence Nightingale). She was in the mould of an independent nurse practitioner blending caring and curing. She seemed to have practised oral rehydration, could reduce fevers, relieve pain and knew the restorative powers of nourishment, rest and direct care. She cared for the elderly, the sick and the dying, successfully dealt with yellow fever and cholera, developed tested and tried her own medicines, (even reportedly curing herself of a cholera attack) and was known in Havanna as 'the yellow woman from Jamaica with the cholera medicine'. Only one book claims her authorship (sometimes disputed).

These exemplary characteristics of a British and a Jamaican role model were entirely lost to us until very recent times.

The hiatus between the Nightingale era and the nursing research renaissance saw some sporadic but important activities which were to have a profound effect on health care and set the stage for different developments in nursing.

After the social upheavals and uprisings of the 1930s in the British Caribbean, the West Indian Royal Commission (Moyne Commission) sent to study the situation in the colonies, made some fundamental recommendations in their report regarding health infrastructure. These were to directly influence the organization of the British West Indian Public Health Training Station in Jamaica (1943) to train public health nurses and inspectors for the British Caribbean. Another related outcome was the inauguration of the University College of the West Indies affiliated to the University of London which opened its doors with a medical school in Jamaica (Mona) in 1948. The University College Hospital with its School of Nursing was a natural development. It is important to note that the purposes of the University Hospital from its incorporation were teaching, research and care.

At that time, nursing was not considered a subject for academic discourse even at the post-basic level. Thus two parallel systems of educating health professionals were perpetuated. However, at about this time nurses began seeking university education where it was available, and attending post-basic nursing programmes in the UK and Canada. Though very few in number, these nurses were mainly assigned to nursing education on return home. Later, nursing service was to also benefit.

In the basic nursing programmes, case histories were introduced and from its inception, the public health nursing field work required a written community project. These may be considered as the very earliest attempts to gather and present data in an organized manner. There were set objectives and an outline to be followed. Nurses had to seek primary sources of information, give factual descriptions, document care given, collect data by interviews, participant observations and careful review of records. Current statistics such as were available had to be utilized. In community projects, public health nursing students would even predict trends based on their analyses and make suggestions for change in aspects of community health care.

The earliest orientation to a systematic methodology seemed to have been an introduction to the epidemiological approach even if in a rudimentary form in the public health nursing programme. Community projects of the period reflected this approach as did the practice of the graduates. A competitive challenge encouraged excellence in the preparation and presentation of these histories and projects. Those adjudged the best by a panel of nurses and doctors earned coveted prizes especially at graduation.

The midwifery programme also provided numerous opportunities for pupils to practice careful, orderly data gathering and factual documentation. It was usually the first introduction to the combined activities of interview, physical examination, description of findings and diagnoses, all recorded in a precise and concise format. Pupil midwives had to explain their findings and support their decisions with data gathered under the watchful scrutiny of experienced qualified midwives. These activities may be considered to be the very earliest attempts at organized data gathering, documentation and use of findings.

Concurrently, the Jamaica General Trained Nurses Association (JGTNA), founded in 1946 and the forerunner of the Nurses Association of Jamaica (NAJ, 1966) was agitating for nursing legislation. A nursing law promulgated in 1951 gave nurses a hitherto unknown measure of control over the education, practice and discipline of nurses.

In 1961 the JGTNA launched its professional magazine *The Jamaican Nurse*. The very first issue carried the article 'Nursing Research and You' written by Miss Mary J. Seivwright, a public health nurse completing a masters programme at Columbia University (Seivwright, 1961). During that year, the first known and published formal nursing research activity with a Jamaican nurse as project director was conducted through the sponsorship of Columbia University and the co-operation of the Ministry of Health. The project director serialized this major event in several issues of *The Jamaican Nurse* during the duration of the project, introducing nurses to a detailed description of various aspects of the research process as they were undertaken. The project was 'Vocational Image of Nurses' and the researcher Miss Mary Seivwright (now Dr Mary Seivwright, Director of the Advanced Nursing Education Unit, University of the West Indies).

It is worthy to note that *The Jamaican Nurse* also published award-winning case studies and community projects. These were due to become important sources of new knowledge regarding local health and illness conditions and their management. In the absence of textbooks which are still almost entirely an imported item, these published reports have been a treasure trove for students and are of historical significance.

Another research activity by Mary Seivwright, 'Factors Affecting Mass Migration of Jamaican Nurses to the United States' was completed and published in 1965. Though pursued to meet academic requirements, the problem chosen was one of extreme relevance and importance. A new phenomenon, nurse migration, began to seriously affect the nursing services of Jamaica. This is the only known study to date that explores the views of a random sample of Jamaican nurses in their adopted environment – in that case, New York. The data underscore the multifaceted nature of the problem. The findings also strongly indicate that the factors need to be addressed simultaneously in order to bring nurse migration 'under reasonable control in the foreseeable future'. The findings of the New York study also support some of the serious concerns repeatedly expressed by nurses in Jamaica. The extent to which these data were utilized by policymakers is unclear. However, several of the recommendations of that study (e.g. reduction of working hours, straight hours (not split) shift system, revision of government and administrative policies regarding post-basic education, promotion, remuneration) were to be slowly implemented at the insistence of the professional organization. It is also quite clear that the failure to consistently and intelligently address the issues identified by migrant nurses in the 1965 study (e.g. working conditions, remuneration, administrative policies) leaves the nursing service of the country in a parlous state today. Twenty-four years later, the problems contributing to migration 'push' factors have intensified, and now affect the attractiveness of nursing as a career choice by prospective students.

During the sixties, there were also functional nursing activity studies conducted in hospitals using the work sampling method. These were done at the behest of the Ministry of Health and made possible by PAHO/WHO. The research team included nurse consultants and local nurse counterparts. The studies addressed utilization of personnel but, although commissioned by government and fully documented reports exist, the extent to which they influenced policy is not quite evident.

A very important study which was to affect nursing education in the British Caribbean was the 1966 survey of 23 schools of nursing directed by Miss R.N. Barrow (now Her Excellency Dr the Hon. Dame Nita Barrow, Barbadian Ambassador to the UN). The survey – a first for the region – was sponsored by the Pan American Health Organization (PAHO/WHO) and instituted among other things the practice of accreditation of schools of nursing.

The single most important development to influence nursing research, was the establishment of post-basic nursing education at the University of the West Indies (UWI) Mona campus. A tripartite agreement between the Government of Jamaica Ministry of Health, PAHO/WHO and the UWI fulfilled this long-awaited expectation of nurses in 1966, and the Advanced Nursing Education Unit (ANEU) began in the Department of Social and Preventive Medicine Medical Faculty, UWI. From its inception, students were required to identify and address a problem of current concern. It was a data gathering and analytic exercise requiring original work and was guided by academic staff.

As the need for research capability increased, the Ministry of Health – Trinidad and Tobago, PAHO/WHO and the UWI at St. Augustine sponsored a month-long research methodology course in September 1968. A major objective was to equip senior nursing personnel in the region with skills to study nursing situations systematically as a basis for plans and programmes to improve nursing service. It was felt that these skills would enable nurses to be more effective on health planning teams. Twenty-four senior nurses from 13 Commonwealth Caribbean countries and Brazil participated. The course was conducted by a PAHO/WHO short-term consultant, assisted by regional nurse advisors and local senior nurses.

In 1971 PAHO/WHO facilitated a Nursing Studies Workshop at the ANEU, UWI (Mona) again providing a short-term consultant. By 1972, the course 'Perspective in Nursing' included a specific introductory unit in research methodology. Theory now occupies some 50 hours in the 11-month certificate programmes. Students also jointly conduct and document at least one study annually. To date, 26 studies have been completed and copies retained in the library. Students are also exposed to research methods in the required psychology course given by the Faculty of Education. Since 1983, the course work for the final year of the BScN includes statistics.

Nurses taking advantage of various other courses in the University, especially prior to the implementation of the BScN, have been engaged in a variety of studies for academic purposes. It is to be observed that these requirements influence nurses to examine current problems systematically and produce a written report that has utility beyond academic purpose.

Nurses have been increasingly engaged in studies providing the data for published reports. Those commissioned by the Ministry of Health or done in the University Hospital do have the distinct possibility of influencing policy, if the project leader pilots the findings into meaningful programmes. A recent island-wide perinatal study engaged many nurses in data collection. The results of these data are being analysed. However, these worthy efforts fall short of nurses themselves initiating, implementing, reporting and publishing studies on their own which have the possibility to influence practice. The research orientation evolving is one in which research helps the nurse to answer questions that are of concern and findings are put to some useful purpose.

From the earliest introduction to research methods inside and outside academia the objective has been to equip nurses for more effective practice – whether they practice as nurse educators, administrators or clinicians. Research is considered a suitable tool in the armamentaria of successful leaders. The problems of functional practice are considered no less important than those of clinical nursing and all are seen as appropriate to enhance the research base of the profession.

Nursing research then is the systematic attempt nurses make to answer any of the numerous testable questions that arise when giving care, teaching care or administering the care system.

The decision to put research methodology in the Certificate Level courses at the ANEU UWI, or year two of the BScN (for registered nurses) is in part based on our urgent need to at least begin a process. The pool of research literate nurses is small and needs to be rapidly expanded. The pool of qualified experienced nurse researchers is even less and has to be improved if there is to be noticeable progress especially in clinical research.

Students at the ANEU have usually completed 10–15 or more years in nursing service and are returning to assume responsible posts if they do not already hold them. Thus their research base needs urgent attention.

## THE HEALTH CARE SYSTEM

The health care system in Jamaica is primarily a government responsibility administered through the Health Ministry, the head of which is a Minister of Health with cabinet status. (The Minister of Health is an elected representative of the people with a political constituency.) Administratively, the chief civil servant is the Permanent Secretary (PS). There is a nursing division headed by a Principal Nursing Officer (PNO). There are nurses responsible for hospital nursing service, nursing education and primary health care nursing. A nursing research officer's post with similar status is yet to be implemented, however the responsibilities of existing senior personnel include research.

The government operates 371 health centres, 12 rural maternity centres, 29 hospitals including 6 specialist institutions (total 6020 beds) and 13 infirmaries. Non-governmental agencies are largely supplied by business, commerce and industry, churches, voluntary agencies and citizens. These include 8 hospitals (284 beds), several extended care facilities for the terminally ill, the elderly and those needing long-term care, numerous clinics which usually serve employees of the sponsoring company or a given clientele in a geographical area.

Four schools of nursing prepare candidates for registration with the Nursing Council by examination. It is interesting to note that one is operated by the Ministry of Health, another by the University Hospital of the West Indies (UHWI), one is in a Community College and another, privately operated, offers a generic degree. All schools use the same clinical areas for practice and there is a student nurses organization embracing all four.

There are three schools of midwifery preparing registered nurses for Nursing Council Midwifery registration examinations. The Ministry of Health also operates programmes to prepare public health nurses, nurse anaesthetists and family nurse practitioners, and offers inservice and continuing education to various categories of nursing personnel. Other programmes currently inactive include basic midwifery, assistant nurse and community health aides. the UHWI operates programmes in critical care, operating theatre techniques, and management of burns. The University of the West Indies (UWI) which is a regional institution serving the English-speaking Caribbean, offers Registered Nurses two certificate courses (nursing education and nursing administration) and a BScN. Nurses also make use of other programmes offered by the UWI and other public and private sector agencies. Thus there are nurses qualified in nutrition, public administration, accounting, health management, community health, epidemiology, mass communication, management studies to name a few.

## HEALTH IN THE JAMAICAN CONTEXT

The population of Jamaica is approximately 2.3 million persons (1982 census) occupying 4411 square miles of largely mountainous terrain with coastal plains. Forty per cent of the people are below the age of 15 and 25% are between the ages of 15 and 24. The number of persons age 65 and over is also increasing. The crude rates for birth (1983) are reported as 26.8 and for deaths (1988) 5.3.

There has been no cholera, yellow fever, small pox and scarlet fever for many decades. Polio, unknown prior to 1957 has been largely brought under control (except for 52 cases in 1982). There are still reported cases of tuberculosis, dengue fever, typhoid, measles, diphtheria and tetanus. The Expanded Programme of Immunization (EPI) is seeking to eliminate these, and the percentage of coverage (as high as 95% in some areas) is very encouraging and illustrates that it can be done. Numerous cases of sexually-transmitted diseases present a pernicious public health problem, and 57 cases of AIDS (May 1988) give great concern.

The leading causes of death are cerebrovascular disease, heart disease and malignant neoplasms. Motor vehicular accidents are a scourge in the younger age group (15–34). The major cause of morbidity is gastroenteritis in children under 5 years of age. The cycle of poverty, illiteracy, unemployment, malnutrition is yet to be broken.

Social factors and life styles which put large sections of the population at high risk, are still the most problematic in health care and clearly the most recalcitrant and impatient of change.

What is health in the Jamaican context? Embracing the Caribbean approach to health through the Caribbean Conference of Ministers Responsible for Health (CCMRH) the following position has been adopted.

> 'It (health) is certainly not just the absence of disease. It is much more. It means that working people are fit and productive and able to acquire and use new skills;
>
> School children are fit and able to benefit from their education and that their physical and mental development have not been permanently impaired by malnutrition in infancy;
>
> 'Every West Indian has the means to either produce or to buy the food he needs;
>
> 'There is dynamic management of the health services;
>
> 'The serious health hazards of the Caribbean environment and the resulting communicable diseases are brought under control;
>
> 'People are emotionally well adjusted individually, in families and as communities and free from dependence on alcohol or tobacco;
>
> 'People have determined for themselves the most important community health problems and are playing their part solving them.'

(Primary Health Care Conference, St Lucia, 1981. CARICOM.)

The second meeting of the CCMRH (1976) named 12 priority health issues that are still problematic:

> 'Poor environmental conditions and resulting communicable diseases;
>
> Insufficient and unsafe water supply, unsanitary excreta disposal and poor food hygiene;
>
> Mothers and children make up 65% of the whole population and have high rates of sickness and death;
>
> Combined malnutrition and diarrhoea disease in children under 2 years of age account for most deaths in this young age group but also for one-fifth to one-third of deaths for all ages;
>
> Twenty to thirty per cent of all deaths in the Caribbean Community are due to communicable diseases and one-third are due to diseases easily prevented by immunization;

Sexually-transmitted diseases are on the increase and tuberculosis remains a problem;

Diabetes and high blood pressure are common, often undetected and uncontrolled;

Mental illness constitutes about one-half of the volume of illness and the mental health services are sadly deficient. Drug abuse falls under this heading;

Diseases of gums and teeth are universal;

All the countries are infected with mosquitoes that transmit dengue and yellow fever;

There is a lack of knowledge and of a sense of responsibility and participation in community health;

There are serious weaknesses in the management of the health services, the availability of trained staff and in the supply and maintenance of health care facilities. The delivery and cost of health care are serious problems.'

(Resolution 4 CCMRH, 1976.)

Every citizen's right to health care is a philosophy espoused in the Caribbean. To realize this each country designs and operates a comprehensive health care system. Certain policies were set in motion even prior to adoption of the Alma-Ata Declaration (1978) embracing the primary health care approach. Thus from the early seventies there was (for example) the Strategy and Plan of Action to Combat Gastroenteritis and Malnutrition (SPACGEM) with specific targets, indictors and time frame for evaluation. While these targets were not achieved in entirety, a process was set in motion which has led to substantial reductions though not elimination of these maladies.

## CURRENT NURSING PROBLEMS

The contemporary and most urgent nursing problem is the manpower resource gap occasioned by nurses leaving the health service for better jobs in the private sector – usually non-nursing – and migration. This pattern has intensified over the past decade. Of particular concern is the loss of experienced nurses with at least two years post-basic education. This loss is most severely felt in all areas of service, management and education. There are many more nurses leaving than entering the profession on an annual basis and the deficit is alarming. This situation leaves both the quality and quantity of nursing care available definitely compromised.

Another serious problem can be explained as the dual epidemiological characteristics of health problems. On the one hand, there are communicable diseases to be eradicated. Though far less a scourge than previously, they can and should be, prevented. Were the necessary resources assigned, this objective could have been realized earlier. On the other hand, lifestyle diseases have overtaken to become the most predominant causes of death. A concerted multidisciplinary and multisectoral primary health care approach is yet to be applied to these. As the population age parameters shift the country still maintains a young age group but must also attend the needs of an ever increasing elderly population with the same intensity given to other age groups.

At every age there is a specific set of risk factors which have to be dealt with and new problems emerge. For example, delinquency can no longer be considered the domain of the courts and correctional services only, but also a major public health problem. An already weakened and tenuous family structure is often unable to provide proper care, security and daily sustenance for three generations under one roof. Thus youths and elders are marginalized and suffer varying degrees of physical and emotional neglect, with dire consequences.

A birth rate of 26.8 represents for Jamaica a substantial reduction in a comparatively short period. However, there have to be far greater efforts to delay first pregnancies among the teenage population, space children, contain family size and further reduce the birth rate.

It would appear that increasing numbers of older persons require hospitalization, need longer hospital stay and sustained support of their recuperative and restorative capacity. As families find it increasingly difficult to retain the elderly in their normal home environment, extended care facilities are essential. This is an area that nurses ought to be addressing in terms of quality of care.

Nurses adhere to traditional ways of care and do not make good use of research findings available to them for the improved practice of nursing. Nurses show more alacrity in implementing research findings of other disciplines, especially when authoritative instructions or decree informs the nurse that a particular line of action (not always explained) is to be taken. Nurses often seek changes based on experiential data or intuition and stop short of the systematic study of many important questions. Although most nurses agree that nursing ought to be a research-based profession this tenet is yet to be aggressively pursued and translated into action. Though many more are seeking to acquire or improve research capabilities there is a serious lag in the numbers of those who actively engage in research as a part of professional practice.

## THE IMPACT OF RESEARCH ON ISSUES OR PROBLEMS

Bearing in mind that a comparative paucity of research exists, that the majority of studies are of a descriptive nature and very few address nursing practice directly there has still been some noticeable work that influenced policy, decision making and change. A few examples will illustrate. The

1965 survey of 23 nursing schools in the Commonwealth Caribbean is considered a watershed in the development of nursing education particularly at basic level. The stated purpose of the project was to 'assess the present training and nursing resources in the British Caribbean as a basis for future planning to improve nursing in all the countries.' (*The Jamaican Nurse*, 4:1:6)

A process was set in motion for curricular changes, improvement in physical facilities and library resources, upgrading nursing tutors and increasing their numbers. These results were to permanently alter the nursing education landscape and were derived from the findings and recommendations of the survey.

The methodology for effecting these changes is instructive.

1. Governments which are responsible for nursing education programmes were not only agreeable but requested PAHO/WHO to undertake the study. Reports then had to be submitted to each government.
2. A regional advisory committee was established. They met with the PAHO/WHO survey team to discuss plans for the study and offer suggestions. The project team added local nurse counterparts in each country. Local nurses then had the opportunity to use the data-gathering tool, participate in interviews, review documents, and inspect physical facilities.
3. A post survey regional seminar of the Regional Advisory Committee, other nursing leaders and the research team was convened to discuss the findings and make recommendations to governments for implementation. PAHO published the survey report and ensured that every seminar participant had a copy. Each school of nursing also received copies.
4. The educational upgrading of the region's tutors began in earnest. Scholarships were provided for tutors to attend the ANEU UWI certificate programmes, one of which was specifically designed for nurse educators.
5. The seminar participants, nursing leaders and ANEU graduates (in a few instances one and the same person) together with selected clinical and administrative nursing colleagues were engaged in the implementation process.
6. There was a time frame as a resurvey was proposed for 1971 and every five years thereafter. If stated, requirements were met to the satisfaction of the survey team and according to set minimum criteria, schools would be accredited.
7. Finally, and most important, the project was led by a highly respected nurse from the region, Miss R. Nita Barrow. She had held posts in nursing education and administration prior to the project, had first hand knowledge of the Caribbean and was a well-known advocate for nursing.

Thus the project was undertaken with the intent of using findings to create change. Nursing leaders were involved from a very early stage. Supportive mechanisms such as the education of tutors to effect meaningful change were put in place. A time frame assisted nurses to prod a somewhat lethargic system into action. PAHO/WHO as the sponsoring agent would retain an active interest in the changes and outcomes and provide assistance with implementation and the resurvey of schools in 1971.

These factors combined in this particular instance to ensure that research findings influenced public policy and brought much desired change in nursing education, the effects of which are still felt today.

The experimental pilot training programme for Community Health Aides (CHA) was initiated in 1967 by the Department of Social and Preventive Medicine, Faculty of Medical Services UWI under the direction of Professor Sir Kenneth Standard, Head of Department, and a multi-disciplinary team in which nurses played a very important role.

Volunteers who had been assisting in clinics were selected and given training to help them function better. This was an urban group located on the perimeter of the UWI and relating to the districts immediately adjacent. The volunteers were persons of limited formal education who were to work under the guidance of registered nurses and registered midwives. They would work in clinics and in the field and have job descriptions. The curriculum, training and evaluation was carried out by experienced nurse educators. The project was established as experimental, carefully developed, guided and evaluated; the process and outcomes documented. Subsequent to the CHA's first year of service (1969) another similar project was piloted in a rural isolated mountainous district with a population of 6000. The Government of Jamaica and Cornell University were now involved. The health staff and citizens selected the candidates who were trained in 1970. The programme targeted malnourished children under 5 years of age and prepared the CHAs to identify these children, weigh and measure them, report to the public health nurse and ensure that they were seen in the clinics. There were special nutritional measures to combat malnutrition and follow-up.

The evaluation indicated that CHAs could be effectively used if trained to deal with specific problems in a particular way and with supervision. This led the Jamaican Government to begin implementation of a CHA programme (1972) in two of the western parishes – Hanover and St James – in the County of Cornwell. A very senior public health nurse was put in charge of this programme which rapidly placed CHAs in all 14 parishes. It was no longer experimental.

A 1973–74 nursing activity study conducted at UHWI by senior nursing staff assisted by a PAHO nurse consultant revealed that student nurses formed the largest group of care givers, especially on night duty. They often worked with minimal or no supervision. Overall they carried 59.3%

of all direct care activities. The investigators concluded that 'a situation in which incompletely qualified persons are providing large amounts of nursing care under minimal or no supervision is potentially dangerous to patients. It is also not conducive to acquiring concepts of care and developing safe appropriate nursing skills.' (Summary of the Nursing Activity Study, UHWI, 1974).

These findings were to strongly support critical changes in nursing education, administration and care. Recommendations to the Board of Management supported by the results of this study eventually led to changes in the apprenticeship system of nursing education; an increase in the number of ward sisters for ward management and staff nurses for clinical care. The responsibility for nursing care was thus shifted from students to professional staff and a more educational approach to nursing curricula undertaken for students.

Disaster Preparedness and Management is a major responsibility in the Caribbean as the area is prone to hurricanes, floods, earthquakes and volcanoes and there are manmade disasters. These destructive forces put whole populations at risk, place immense strain on fragile economies, destroy the agricultural base of the countries, stretch the capacity of the health care system and the resilience of the people to withstand, survive and start again.

All health disciplines need to be alert to disaster preparedness and management as health personnel are essential to the response capability of a country. In Jamaica concern was expressed at what was perceived as inadequate curricular attention by the health disciplines to the concept and strategies of disaster preparedness

Under the auspices of the Pan Caribbean Disaster Preparedness and Prevention Project a Caribbean workshop was convened in Antigua 1982. Managerial level personnel from the health disciplines of both Government and non-governmental agencies met for discussion and simulation exercises. The curricular concern gathered momentum and the Project Director commissioned a study which was to ascertain 'the extent to which disaster preparedness is included in programmes of health personnel offered by the UWI and other educational and training institutions in Jamaica' (Marshall-Burnett and Pinnock, 1983). The study embraced 28 programmes in 14 institutions serving 10 health disciplines occupying 22 job categories in the health services as well as private sector. The convenience sample included at least one senior educator in each programme who completed the specially developed questionnaire and was interviewed. Where available, curricular material was also examined. The study aroused much interest. Interviewees spoke freely of their concerns and their desire to be better informed so that they could teach the subject. They also had need for materials and teaching aids as well as other resources and hoped that the findings of the study would receive attention. Participants offered suggestions regarding appropriate ways to deal with the subject matter. Findings indicated that only 12 of 28 programmes had any content on the subject. Two to 16 hours were allotted and the material was superficial. Respondents urged a common core of information for all disciplines with job specific responsibilities added. They felt a multidisciplinary 'training of trainers' programme was necessary and simulation exercises. Nurses were the largest group, occupying several job categories in primary, secondary and tertiary care. The study report was submitted to the Project Director in June 1983. As a consequence two workshops were convened in September 1983 and February 1984 to assist educators in the preparation of curricular content and use of simulation methodology. Sponsored by PAHO, the Ministry of Health and the Office of Disaster Preparedness and Emergency Relief Coordination (ODIPERC) Jamaica, there were 23 educators at each workshop.

*The Disaster Preparedness and Management Curriculum for Health Professionals, Jamaica 1984*, published by PAHO is the account of the workshop activities and serves as a guide to all programmes. The subject matter is now a part of the curricula of the various health disciplines. There is a core course for all sections and job category information. It is important to note that the respective educational institutions willingly released their staff to participate and the educators undertook to implement necessary change even where course work was already tightly scheduled. The promptness with which the Project Director responded, convinced participants of the attention given to their views and opinions.

A current example of nursing research influencing public policy is one of great importance and has major implications for the future of the profession.

Five members of the 1984–85 class of Registered Nurses pursuing certificate courses at the ANEU UWI expressed grave concern regarding what they considered a drastic reduction in the number of students in the basic three-year professional nursing programmes. They felt it was a problem worth investigating in fulfilling their academic requirements of the completion and presentation (oral and written) of a study.

These early investigators gleaned information which revealed that one school of nursing has suffered a 46.4% decline in the number of applicants during the five-year period 1977–82. Schools also indicated that some candidates admitted to the programme failed to commence the programme. This was particularly noticeable in a school that made special effort to attract male candidates. The Nursing Council recorded a 30% decline in the number of Jamaican-trained nurses taking the registration examination between 1973 and 1984.

The Ministry of Health took the position that the already comparatively modest academic entrance requirements set by Nursing Council were too high and constituted a deterrent to prospective applicants. They pointed to overall low national results in the General Certificate of Education (GCE) and Caribbean Examination Council (CXC) Examinations particularly in compulsory subjects required by Council. However, it was observed that there were no shortages of qualified applicants for medical school where the available places were sought after by more than twice as many applicants. Over many years none of these applicants considered nursing an acceptable alternative or second choice as a career.

The ANEU students concluded that the young people who were staying away from nursing had good reasons for so doing, and admission requirement was not the critical factor in the decline of applicants to nursing school. Nurse educators repeatedly pointed out that when general education requirements were less than the Nursing Council's current minimum, students experienced great difficulty and remedial work had to be undertaken. This created hardships for students and teachers alike. Post-basic education was also being jeopardized by low secondary educational level. They were therefore not in favour of reduced entry requirements.

The NAJ strongly believed that the problems associated with the increasing number of resignations from the service were also a major deterrent to young persons entering the profession.

The five ANEU students having discussed these points therefore designed a study which sought to answer the question: 'What factors are reported as influencing the choice of nursing as a career by fifth-form students in selected Jamaican High Schools.'

Fifth-form students were the target population on the basis that they were at that point in the general education system where they would be making career choices, pursuing the qualifications which would ensure entry for their chosen career and would frankly and openly share their views. (Factors influencing High School Student, ANEU, 1985.)

The accessible population was 1098 fifth-form students from five co-educational secondary schools in three parishes with urban and rural representation. A random sample of 100 students was chosen (20 from each school). The students' ages ranged from 14 (one student) to 19 (one student) with a mean age of 16.2 years. There were 64 females and 36 males, reasonable reflecting the sex ratio in fifth form. The data-gathering instrument was a specially developed nine-item questionnaire with open and closed ended questions examined for content validity but not pretested. The instrument was administered in each school by one investigator to all 20 students at one sitting.

All students were preparing for either the GCE (17 students) or the CXC (27 students) or doing subjects in both examinations (56 students); 59 of the students (33 girls and 26 boys) were pursuing subjects which if successfully completed would make them eligible for nursing school. Students indicated that the factors influencing their career choice included:

good salary, fringe benefits and promotion
financial security and stable employment
opportunity to travel and meet people

parental influence
service to people
possibility of working independently
friends, guidance counsellors and advertisements

When asked to indicate three career choices in order of preference, health-related careers were the most popular choices given by the 93 students who answered the question. Medicine was the most frequent with 19 choices and nursing next with 16 choices. No male student chose nursing; neither did any student, male or female, from an urban school which caters for the upper class; nor did any student from one rural school consider nursing a first or second choice. An urban school with a nursing programme on its campus fared no better than another urban school without a nursing programme in terms of nursing being a first career choice. Altogether there were five first choices from three schools, none of the schools having more than two first choices. The school with the nursing programme on its campus had the largest number of second choices and accounted for 11 of the 16 choices.

Fourteen of these 16 students indicated that they had relatives and friends who were nurses. They also gave humanitarian reasons as the major basis of their choice and although 4 stated that upward social mobility was possible not one mentioned remuneration as a reason for their choice.

Of the 77 students who did not name nursing among their career choices 74 gave their reasons. The major one advanced were categorized as personal and idiosyncratic such as inability to deal with sick people and aversion to blood. The second category of reasons named were socio-economic factors such as salary, fringe benefits, inconvenient hours. Thirty of the 74 students gave a reason in this category as their first cause for not choosing nursing as a career. It is interesting to note that while many students stated that the nursing profession was important and essential they also stated that nurses were 'unfairly treated'. This image was persistent and unattractive. No student made reference to academic requirements as a reason for not choosing or for that matter choosing nursing as a career.

These findings were used by the NAJ in discussion with Ministry officials to support the general education criteria set by Nursing Council, to argue against any reduction in academic criteria and to urge a wider study from which more confident generalizations could be made. The five-school sample was not considered broad enough, given the very large secondary school population island wide. The results, however, were both instructive and interesting.

Nursing personnel in the Ministry proceeded with its own study using a larger sample but the Nursing Council undertook an island-wide study.

Preliminary reports would indicate that fifth formers in the island do not differ considerably in their choices and opinions from the five-school sample investigated earlier.

In the meantime Nursing Council decided to temporarily relax its mathematics requirement in terms of the grade required to test the influence on intake, because nursing schools were having great difficulty in attracting candidates. Although the number of candidates to one school is said to have increased 100% it must be shown that no school currently has even 50% of its original class size in either first, second or third year. There has been no avalanche of applicants.

In 1988, four ANEU students designed a study 'Views of Third-year Nursing Students regarding the Nursing Profession'. All 99 third-year nursing students in three schools of nursing (one school had no third-year class) is the sample; 65 of these students had more than the Nursing Council's minimum requirements. Of the 99 only 2 considered the entrance requirements too high and 7 said that mathematics was not needed. This study is not yet completed.

The fifth-form study re career choices done by new investigators as part of academic requirements began the process of closely examining a major problem. Prior to this study there were beliefs, conjecture and experience. Systematic investigation has uncovered some important factors, influenced a stay of precipitate action and formed the background to islandwide studies. Summary of this study given at a meeting with Ministry officials generated much interest and not a little surprise that within academia, nurses as beginning researchers are concerned with problems faced in daily work.

Already there is evidence that the Government is looking at the physical environment of its nursing school and has announced plans to relocate the school in another building. Attention to the infrastructure of institutions and agencies providing clinical practice is also being undertaken. A major clinical facility which was temporarily removed from the suitable list of agencies for clinical practice is now restored.

Other suggestions regarding pre-nursing courses and suitable general education preparation of prospective candidates are also under consideration. Applicants to basic nursing education programmes need to have general secondary education which contributes to professional education. This is critical to the practice of nursing. It is far too important a matter to be the subject of controversy, speculation or manipulation. The scientific method is to help us increase our knowledge and our information regarding questions that impinge on practice. The findings of these studies will be available to government to guide them in policy making which will have both short-and long-term implications for the education and practice of the profession.

## CONCLUSION

Research will be of no value to the profession if its final resting place is the splendid obscurity of library shelves. Research has to be used by persons who find it meaningful, interesting and relevant to the problems they confront. Also research has to be understood often in greater detail than the edited version a publication offers. This may mean correspondence with the researcher. It is people therefore who have to activate the use of research findings by ensuring that after careful evaluation, practice is indeed guided by what is available. It may be then that researcher and consumers have to form a network from the earliest stages of conceptualization of a problem and work together in ways that are helpful so that having been engaged in the research process the outcomes are not alien but part of the consumers' frame of reference. Such collaboration will no doubt demystify the undertaking and bring the researcher in the arena where action takes place. It will not only build bridges of understanding and facilitate communication but contribute to the translation of theory into practice. No one said it was easy, but it is possible.

## REFERENCES

Alternatives in the Delivery of Health Services. St Lucia Workshop Report 1971. Department of Social and Preventive Medicine, UWI Mona.

A Report of the Survey of Schools in the Caribbean (1966) PAHO/WHO, Washington.

Factors Influencing Migration of Registered Nurses from Jamaica to the United States of America 1978–1983. (1985) ANEU, UWI Mona.

Factors Influencing High School Students in their choice of Nursing as a Career (1985) ANEU, UWI, Jamaica.

Marshall-Burnett, Syringa and Pinnock, Milton (1983) 'Disaster Preparedness in Curricula of Health Professionals.' Pan Caribbean Disaster Preparedness Project Antigua. PAHO/WHO, Barbados.

Merton, Robert (1958) address to the 41st ANA Convention, ANA, NY.

Omawale and Subaran Sonia (1983) The Caribbean Community Health Management. The State of the Art Institute of Social and Economic Research UWI, Jamaica (internal document).

Summary of the Findings of the Nursing Activity Study and the Use of Student Nurses in the Clinical Area (1974) UHWI, Jamaica.

Report of the Proceedings of the Second Caribbean Conference of Ministers Responsible for Health (CCMRH) 1976. CARICOM Secretariat, Guyana.

Report of the Primary Health Care Conference St Lucia 1981. CARICOM Secretariat, Guyana.

Seivwright, Mary J. (1961) Nursing research and you. *The Jamaican Nurse* 1:1:19 Vocational Image of Public Health Nurses. (1961, 1962) *The Jamaican Nurse* 1:2:35 2:2:32 2:3:8.

Seivwright, Mary (1965) Factors affecting mass migration of Jamaican nurses to the United States. *The Jamaican Nurse* 5:2:8.

Views of Third-year Nursing Students regarding the Nursing Profession (1988) ANEU UWI, Jamaica.

# CHAPTER SIX

# Nursing research in Spain: present situation and future expectations

*Myriam Ovalle Bernal*

This chapter has been prepared as an overview of nursing and nursing research in Spain. It is not intended to be exhaustive.

Although existing documents claim that nursing research in Spain is scarce and at an early stage, the last decade is marked by growing advancement. Many factors have influenced this rapidly expanding area, but the most significant was the placement of basic education at university level in 1977. Another important issue during the last five years was the primary health care approach. It provided a new frame of reference for nursing practice, education and research that influenced the perspectives of nursing research and will give direction to nursing research activities in the future.

## GENERAL INFORMATION

The major part of the Spanish territory is situated in the Iberian Peninsula and also includes the Balearic and Canary Islands. The total land area is $504750$ km$^2$. It is considered a mountainous country, since 18% of the territory has an altitude of more than 1000 m.

The census in 1988 recorded 39.2 million inhabitants. The density is 77.66 inhabitants per square kilometre, with the majority living in big cities. The population growth rate has been constant during the last decades, around 1%. The maximum growth rates of the population coincide with the decades of economic development: 1920–30 and 1960–70. There is a rapid increase of the 65+ age group and a decline in the 0–14 group.

As in most European countries , the main causes of illness and death in Spain are cardiovascular conditions, malignant tumours and accidents. It has been calculated that between 10 to 15% of all deaths are attributable in one way or another to smoking and more than 4% to alcohol consumption and drug dependence. Infant mortality (15.2) is similar to that of developed countries and the decline in infant mortality is considerable. The maternal mortality rate (0.13), also shows a declining rate but is higher in some autonomic regions.

The Spanish population faces a number of changes likely to be irreversible in the near future, such as changing patterns in family composition, increase in the number of divorces, unemployment (specially of young people and women), changing role of women, increase in the number and proportion of the elderly, concentration of population in certain areas and decline of birth rates. In general, the economic crises, the demographic, epidemiological and social changes in the population increase the need for health and social services. Therefore, the Government is confronted with the challenge to adjust the health policies and the health system in order to provide the appropriate health services in the near future.

## EVOLUTION OF THE HEALTH SYSTEM

In the 1940s the health system was developed around a strong public sector within the social security system. There is also a private health sector providing service. Although the National Health Institute (INSALUD) covers 85% of the population, its available financial resources are only 70% of the total resources of the national health sector, and it only owns a quarter of the total number of hospital beds in the country. This is a problem that has been solved through agreements with the other institutions of the public and private health institutions.

There are certain inequalities in health care coverage. For example, the 3.2% of the population with low income as well as to 2% of the population with medium–low income are unprotected and are not covered by the public health services. In 1986, the Parliament passed the General Health Bill which is based on the principles and concepts of primary health care. This bill is oriented towards health care services for the whole population. The development of this bill calls for a change in attitudes of policy-makers and health professionals and better use of the available resources, especially during this time of economic constraints. It also requires reorientation of professional education and research to produce new knowledge to improve the quality of health services and the quality of life for all the population.

The General Health Bill established principles to ensure the access of all the population to the health services and reduce inequalities. A great deal of effort and willingness will be required on the part of health authorities to distribute the financial resources based on the principle of equity in order to guarantee access to health services all over the Spanish territory. Although the process has begun, it can be said that the health services are still focused mainly on disease rather than on promotion of health and prevention of illness. Emphasis is on individuals rather than on community or groups at risk.

## PRESENT SITUATION OF THE NURSING PROFESSION AND MAIN PROBLEM AREAS

### Nursing services

The Report of the National Conference on Nursing and Primary Health Care, held in 1983 points out that nursing services, as an integral part of the health system, must be organized according to the same pattern.

During the last ten years the health system experienced an initial change towards better co-ordination of the health services, decentralization and expansion of covered population based on the principles of primary health care. But it is also evident that the lack of political willingness to accelerate the change, the instability of the economic environment, and the negative reactions from the health professions, have limited progress.

Although nurses have been prepared for comprehensive health care for individuals, families and communities, most of them follow the medical model and their activities concentrate on the care of the sick individual rather than on the promotion of health and preventive actions. Some nurses have progressively assumed primary health care functions, specially for groups with chronic health problems. In some autonomic governments nurses have received legislative support to fulfil these functions, although it is quite limited in the promotion of health and the prevention of disease.

A Royal Decree (521/1987) of the Ministry of Health introduced an initial change for the advancement of autonomy in the administration of nursing services. It is established that nursing divisions be at the same level as the medical and administrative divisions in each hospital. These three division chiefs make up the governing board, sharing responsibility for the administration of the hospital as a whole.

In the area of primary health care and community health there is an urgent need for regulatory policies and clarification of the place of nursing administration in these services.

At national, autonomic and local levels of health administration there is a lack of nurses in executive positions. Most nurses at these levels are in advisory positions, usually directly responsible to a physician or an administrator without direct access to officers at higher levels. Participation of nurses in the total health care planning is limited to decisions affecting nursing.

In 1988 the Minister of Health appointed a nurse to its advisory group, and another nurse has been appointed to a section of the General Division for Health Planning of the Ministry of Health. Others in the Primary

Health Care and Hospital Divisions of the Health Institute (INSALUD) are in an advisory capacity.

## Nursing manpower

The General Council of Nurses reported 147 000 as the total number of registered nurses in 1988, wih a ratio of about one nurse to 300 persons. The ratio is highest in the large cities. It is considered that, according to the existing ratio of nurses to population, there is not a quantitative shortage of nurses. However, a qualitative shortage exists regarding the lack of specialists in areas such as community nursing, nursing service administration, geriatric nursing and mental health-psychiatric nursing. These specialties have been approved recently and still are in the process of developing the curriculum.

In Spain it is difficult to find reliable data or studies about the nursing profession: numbers, distribution, functions, use of personnel, trends in unemployment or underemployment, or the number of schools that have revised the curriculum towards primary health care of community-based training. This situation requires research and prospective studies for developing sound nursing manpower planning based on health needs of the population, the role and education of the generalist/specialist nurse within our health care system.

In February 1988 a research project along these lines was proposed by the General Council of Nursing. The main purpose of this project is to study the nursing manpower situation within the country and to use the data as a base to develop prospective actions needed in nursing service, nursing education, nursing administration and nursing research. A joint effort by the Ministry of Health, Ministry of Education and the General Council of Nursing is expected to make possible this national research project.

There is also a need to establish permanent information systems for collection of data on nurse manpower in the health services and education at national, regional and local levels.

## Nursing education

*Basic nursing education.* Nursing leaders recognize that the most significant step towards the advancement in nursing education was the educational legislation passed in 1977. This legislation placed basic nursing education at the first cycle of the university education system in the country with a three-year program leading to a Nursing Diploma (Diplomado en Enfermeria). Directives for development of the university nursing programs were established by the Ministry of Education. In the curriculum new content was introduced on the nursing process, nursing models and theories, social and behavioural sciences, geriatric nursing, mental health nursing, public health and research.

During the 1977–87 decade nursing education experienced the most challenging development and progress in a short time. However, the present situation of nursing education demands new efforts to improve the quality of basic nursing education, specially in the following areas of concern identified by the author in 1984.

Out of the 90 university schools of nursing, 17 belong to the public universities. The other 73 are academically dependent on public universities and financially on private institutions, the National Health Institute or autonomic health institutes. An assessment of the quality of education provided in the nursing schools has not yet been carried out.

Clinical experience in community nursing and primary health care is only provided by a few schools because the structure for primary health care services is not fully developed and the faculty teaching in these areas do not have sound preparation in community nursing or primary health care. Thus, an unacceptable gap exists between theory and practice.

Most of the schools place emphasis on content without relating all the subjects to a conceptual frame of reference for curriculum design, or taking into account the student's learning process and the use of an active methodology.

Very few schools of nursing are directed by nurses, the majority are directed by physicians. As a result, most of the curricula follow medical models instead of nursing models, and the focus on treatment of disease persists.

Since the second cycle of our university system leading to a bacca- laureate degree has not been developed for nursing, the nursing faculty does not have access to advanced nursing education leading to an academic degree. This factor is an obstacle to ensuring the quality of basic university nursing education and to further preparation for the research endeavour.

It is recognized that there is a qualitative shortage of nursing faculty with advanced training in clinical areas, nursing education, administration and research.

All these problem areas call for strategic planning and future action in nursing education.

After ten years of nursing education within the university setting and the social, economic, political, legal and educational changes in the country, a critical analysis and modifications are needed in university education. This is taking place under the provision of the General Law for University Education. The Ministry of Education has appointed a Commission of

Health Professions (including nurses, physicians and others), representing the practising professions, educators and authorities from the Ministries of Health and Education. Each professional group formed a subcommission to analyse the current situation and make proposals. The nursing subgroup worked during 1977, and presented a proposal that is under discussion in schools of nursing and the General Council of Nursing. It is expected that the Ministry of Education will take the suggestions of the groups into account before reaching the final decision about the new General Directives for basic studies. These Directives include minimum requirements to assure the quality of education needed to prepare a nurse generalist to function autonomously in relation to the changing needs and new trends in the sociopolitical environment, the health sector and the health of the population, and have enough flexibility for creativity and pursuit of excellence in each university school of nursing.

In this independent role the nurse will be responsible for planning, implementation and evaluation of nursing care with the participation of individuals, families, groups and communities. Therefore, the nurse will need sound preparation in managerial and research aspects to be able to function in an interdisciplinary setting in a responsible partnership, and to introduce changes in nursing practice oriented to primary health care.

The new Project of Directives to develop plans for basic nursing education states that the first cycle of nursing education should prepare a generalist nurse able to meet the health needs of individuals and groups taking into account sociocultural patterns, resources available in the country, existing legislation and the nurse's own personal development.

Once the diploma in nursing has been obtained, the option exists for continuing studies in a second cycle of nursing, which is the equivalent to a baccalaureate degree. A proposal for obtaining the official recognition of this degree has already been raised with the Ministry of Education and it is now pending approval. It is hoped that these new directives will serve as a cornerstone for the legal support needed to change the present situation.

*Post-basic nursing education.* The specialties have been regulated by the Government in the Royal Decree (922/1987) of the Ministry of Health. This decree creates seven nursing specialties: obstetric-gynaecological nursing (midwifery), paediatric nursing, mental health nursing, community health nursing, medical/surgical nursing, geriatric nursing and nursing management and administration. These specialties will be developed in university teaching units supervised by schools of nursing. There is a provision to establish a National Council of Nursing Specialties, as a consultant body to the Ministries of Education and Health. It has to be pointed out that for the first time there will be specialties in nursing management and administration, community health nursing and geriatric nursing at the university level. The preparation for these specialty areas was offered before this Decree as continuing education programs with great variety of length and content.

## DEVELOPMENT AND PERSPECTIVES OF NURSING RESEARCH

Wihin this context of continuous and accelerated sociopolitical, economic and health changes, nursing has become aware of the need to generate knowledge and to use research to solve nursing problems.

Since the mid-70s emphasis has been on development of nursing education. Nursing leaders have worked towards the objective of integrating basic and post-basic nursing studies within the educational system of the country at university level. This emphasis will continue in the next decade in order to develop baccalaureate and doctoral education programmes. Although the emphasis has been on education, the increasing interest in research is concurrent with the beginning of basic nursing university education in 1977. Nurses have perceived that research is a basic requirement for responsible professional practice and to improve the quality of nursing education.

The Government has initiated a reorientation of the health system which is still considered insufficient to reduce the existing gap between the health needs of the people and the resources available to meet the targets of Health for All. These resources should include research capability, knowledge and support of a national health research policy.

Nurses have the responsibility, more than any other health profession, to accelerate the development of primary health care strategy in the country, but at the same time they recognize that they are not sufficiently prepared for this task. Therefore, nursing research should be focused on areas such as healthy life styles, community participation in health care, identification of health needs of groups at risk and development of new models to provide nursing care within the primary health care system.

Another aspect to consider in our situation is the existing controversy between the objectives of the health system and health professionals' roles. Given the economic situation of the health sector characterized by instability and limited financial resources to face the increasing demand for comprehensive health care services, nursing practice as an autonomous profession has been questioned, specially by physicians. Therefore, new roles and new models to provide nursing care should be explored and developed.

Autonomy is a key concern of professional nurses, particularly in primary health care. How to apply this concept in nursing practice, education and research is still unclear. The main problem remains in our legislation for nursing practice where there are few activities that the nurse can perform without delegation from physicians. Thus, those who have the responsibility for administration of nursing practice must cope with the problem of applying obsolete legislation to new functions accepted by nurses in its new role of primary health care.

In the minds of some health professionals and laymen, nursing functions often look like medical ones. This leads to confusion about what distinguishes nursing from medicine. Therefore, research is urgently needed to progress towards a more autonomous practice characterized by identity, independence and authority based on theory and rationale for nursing practice.

## Nursing research manpower

In the recent Report on National Debates about Health for All Targets and Implications for the Nursing Profession (Ministry of Health, 1987), there was agreement within the nurse participants that there is a shortage of nurse researchers in Spain. The concept of nursing research manpower used in this context refers not only to the number of nurses able to design, conduct and report research work, but also to the number of research nurse educators, nurse administrators, nurse clinicians, as well as the level of expertise of each of them.

Of the 147000 registered nurses, 60000 graduated from the Sanitary Technical Assistants (ATS) programmes existing before 1977. This programme did not include research in its curriculum content. Approximately 87000 graduated from the three-year programme established in 1977 leading to a university diploma or from a complementary programme for ATS to reach the level of a university diploma. This programme included basic research content in the curriculum for *Diplomados en Enfermeria* (first university cycle).

In Spain, nurses have identified the need for baccalaureate (*Licenciatura*) level of education as an urgent need to improve the quality of nursing services and nursing education. A project for development of this second cycle within the university system was developed and approved by the 9th Commission established in 1987 by the Council of Universities. Nevertheless, the university authorities are delaying the decision about this level of education for nurses. Specialties recently approved do not lead to an academic degree. Within our educational system, this kind of education is considered at the university level, but in a special way developed for physician specialties.

Very few nurses have earned nursing baccalaureate, masters of doctoral degrees outside the country. The author estimates a total of ten nurses with a masters degree. Therefore, Spain has relatively few nurses with advanced research training. It does not constitute adequate research manpower, specially if we consider the total population (39.2 million) the extent of the territory (504750 km$^2$), the number of registered nurses (147000), the number of schools of nursing (90), the complexity of the health services (hospitals and health centres), the local, autonomic and national levels of administration, the extensive coverage of the population by the public health system and the expected improvement in quality of nursing care. A present, there are no full-time nurse researchers employed by the educational or health institutions, or full-time nurse research consultants. In this regard policies should be adopted to promote the employment of nurse researchers in educational and health institutions and to enhance the nursing research manpower to ensure the nursing contribution to meet the people's health needs.

## Education for nursing research

*Basic education.* Formal education for nursing research was introduced in 1977 when basic education was placed at a university level. The number of credits for elementary research preparation was integrated in the Directives from the Ministry of Health within a course labelled 'Fundamental Nursing'. It also included preparation in statistics and epidemiology. Although this change was favourable to the development of nursing research, a lack of well-prepared nursing faculty has been a limitation. Data from a survey conducted by the General Council of Nursing on Nursing Research between 1933 and 1988 evidenced that the majority of professors of basic education programmes (75%) have completed only introductory courses in research and that they don't have access to university advanced preparation in research. This problem is aggravated by the fact that many schools (70%) don't allow the nursing faculty time for research. The workload includes only teaching and supervisory activities. Only three university schools of nursing reported an institutional research plan with priorities developed by the nursing faculty.

*Post-basic education.* The development of post-basic nursing education has not progressed at the same pace as basic education. It has taken ten years after the change of basic programmes in 1977 to structure the education of nursing specialists at university level.

As already mentioned, the legislation on nursing specialties was passed in July 1987. In this level of education, the research component should be one of the essential parts of the specialists' curriculum. If the nurse specialist is expected to be a leader and an expert in the appropriate field of specialization, a sound preparation is needed to use research in solving nursing and health problems, to develop authoritative decision-making based on research findings, to identify significant problems in settings where nursing care is delivered, to conduct research into these problems and apply the findings to nursing practice.

*Continuing education.* Continuing education programmes in research have been the main resource for nursing research preparation. Most of them have introductory courses to research methodology and statistics offered by a diversity of institutions, such as scientific associations, university schools of nursing, nursing colleges and some private institutions which offer nursing service administration programmes. Some of these programmes require the development of a research project.

A survey conducted by the author on continuing nursing education in 1988, showed that 40 of the 52 nursing colleges offer nursing courses in three main areas: primary health care, new trends and developments in nursing and nursing service administration. Research was not included as a priority for continuing education. Nevertheless, there is an increasing demand from nurses motivated to initiate research or to follow advanced research courses.

The need for a national plan for continuing education and co-ordination was obvious. Consequently, a national project based on health needs of the population, nurses' needs to assume new roles and responsibilities and trends in the health care system has been initiated by the General Council of Nursing. Research will be part of this national programme; the purpose is to promote the development of nursing research and give opportunities to motivated nurses to be prepared for research endeavours.

## Funding for nursing research

The development of research not only depends upon the availability of experts, but also on financial support. In Spain research funding is available from four main sources: Government research funds; national autonomic and local health service funds; university research funds and private agencies and foundations.

Within the national context funding is very limited for nurses researchers due to:

Funds available for research in the health field are allocated mainly to biomedical research.

One of the requirements to have access to available funds for research from the Ministry of Health or from university settings is to hold a baccalaureate degree (*Licenciatura*), which is not yet developed in the nursing system of education.

On the other hand, most of the agencies, foundations or institutions with available funds for nursing research allocate these resources mainly for projects to developing countries. They do not take into account that in nursing research Spain is at a level similar to the developing areas.

With the integration of Spain into the European Community a new path has been opened to finance nursing projects through the health programmes of the European Community such as the Euro-Cancer Programme, the Aids Programme and the Geriatric Programme and also through the Erasmus Programme which promotes an international network between European universities.

## Production of scientific endeavour

Analysis of scientific production in nursing described by the author in Reports on Development of Nursing Research in Spain 1983–1986 underline the following aspects:

Prior to 1977 nursing research production was scarce. Nurses used to participate in medical research, mainly gathering data, and not throughout the whole research process. Therefore, nurses usually didn't appear as researchers in those publications,

The initiation of nursing university education constituted a point of departure for a growing development in scientific production. The introduction of research in the basic curriculum was a motivating factor for nursing faculty to look for better preparation and engagement in research.

During the last decade nursing research has been the result of personal initiatives of nurse researchers. A few health institutions, such as hospitals or health centres, or educational institutions (university, schools of nursing) developed a research nursing plan. A survey of Nursing Research between 1983 and 1988, already cited, shows that only five university schools of nursing have defined priorities for nursing research to be assumed as institutional responsibility. Few hospital nursing departments have initiated a research institutional plan. Research in the field of community nursing is mainly a joint effort of local government and nurses working at district levels or in health centres. The research reports presented at national nursing congresses are very seldom published due to lack of finances. During the last five years nursing faculty from 14 schools of nursing have engaged in research regardless of the lack of institutional interest or available facilities. From 1983 to 1988 research reported by 14 schools of nursing has been done in the area of community nursing (36%), medical and surgical nursing (32%), geriatric nursing (16%), nursing administration (6%), maternal and child nursing (4%), mental health (4%) and nursing education (2%).

Nurse researchers are giving special attention to the nursing care of patients with cancer problems. This is the second cause of mortality in Spain. On the other hand, in the national context and the European Community, research in this area is considered a priority. Most of these studies deal with management of patients. There are few studies in the preventive area of cancer or in the promotion of a healthy life style in order to decrease the cancer risk factors. Some of the nursing problems studied are in the domain of nurses' attitudes to terminal patients, towards pain in cancer patients, psychological aspects of suffering in cancer patients.

An example of the initial stage of the nursing research endeavour and growing interest of nurse researchers in patients with cancer problems is the study on Nurses' Attitudes towards Pain in Cancer Patients conducted by Apilanez in 1983. The summary of the report points out that pain is one of the main problems of cancer patients which nurses must deal with to provide adequate nursing care. The sample was composed by 15 nurses providing direct nursing care to cancer patients in a nursing unit of a teaching hospital. Observation was used to identify nurses' attitudes. Recorded observation described the following attitudes:

1.  When patients requested a pain-reliever, nurses didn't identify the cause of pain.
2.  When medical instructions existed for the administration of analgesic drugs, nurses administered it to the patient without questioning the origin of the patient's pain.
3.  Nurses assumed that only drugs would relieve the pain. Other nursing interventions regarding psychological support were not used to deal with or relieve the patient's pain.
4.  Nurses experienced anxiety when pain-reliever drugs didn't rapidly produce the desired effects, and the patient asked for another pain-reliever. In these cases nurses urged the physician to administer pain-reliever drugs or tranquilizers of greater strength or frequency.

Based on these findings, it was concluded:

> The need for further exploration of the cause of pain in cancer patients to enhance the nurses knowledge on this matter.
> The need for better communication and interaction with patients to identify the cause and kind of pain.
> The need to use psychological approaches to deal with patient anxiety and pain as well as nurses' anxiety.
> The need to assess the patient's needs and develop an individualized nursing care plan.

Since this study was conducted in a teaching hospital, nurse teachers, nurse practitioners of the cancer unit and nursing students have developed projects in relation to the identified needs in order to enhance the nurses' knowledge about pain in cancer patients, psychological approaches to deal with anxiety and pain and the improvement of nursing care plans and records. Although the study was considered as an initial development in cancer nursing research, the findings have had an impact on the nursing practice and nursing education of the teaching hospital.

A strategy initiated in some schools of nursing to enlarge the scientific production, is the co-operation of practitioners, faculty and students to identify nursing problems and develop joint research projects. This strategy has been used mainly in community nursing and primary health care research.

Nursing studies conducted in community health and primary health care settings are contributing to the identification of nursing care needs and the the development of nursing care models to provide nursing care to specific groups at risk, such as diabetic or hypertensive patients.

As an example of the research production, it can be observed that in the International Nursing Research Congress that took place in Madrid 1983, Spanish nurse researchers presented 16 papers and 26 posters sessions on a wide variety of topics. This type of international meeting is of special importance in providing a forum which allows nurse scholars to develop an international network, increase the knowledge and use of research and identify issues and opportunities for sharing nursing research. These international events also increase the awareness of the need for nursing research and motivate other nurses to initiate research.

The Nursing Unit of the World Health Organization, Regional Office for Europe, developed a multinational study on People's Needs for Nursing Care with participation of eleven European countries. Spanish nurses did not have the opportunity to participate in it, but the study has been presented by some of the authors in several national congresses and has motivated nurses interested in research activities. This multinational European study constitutes another example of networking useful not only for nursing research development, but also for nursing leadership development in research areas.

In general, there is a need for more expertise in research and leadership development to enhance an accelerated research production. Developing national and international networking for nursing research could be of great help to increase the level of expertise of the research community and the needed leadership to initiate changes and promote research work.

## Dissemination of nursing research

The increase of nursing research raises problems of dissemination of findings, and other information related to research in process. The survey of nursing research 1983–88 suggested that dissemination and communication of research findings and research projects require the use of more adequate channels than the existing ones, making the research more readily available to nurses within the academic and health contexts. During the last decade the number of nursing publications, specially nursing journals, has increased. The General Council of Nurses publishes a quarterly journal

'*New Nursing*' for all nurses in the country; 32 of the 52 provincial colleges of nursing have a journal and the other 20 publish a newspaper or bulletin to be sent to the nurses in the province; these publications very seldom include research reports.

Publications from scientific nursing societies like the Cancer Society include research projects and summaries of nursing research reports. During the last five years research was disseminated mainly through national congresses, workshops and seminars, but in general remained unpublished due to lack of financial resources.

## Primary health care and nursing research

Nurses are aware that the primary health care strategy in the European region presents a new frame of reference for the future development of nursing practice, education, administration and research. In 1987 the authorities from the Ministry of Health and the General Council of Nursing, as well as autonomic governments and colleges of nursing, organized 214 nursing forums throughout the 17 autonomic regions of the country. In these forums nurses identified the need to develop research in order to be able to fulfil the new role of the nurse in primary health care and contribute to the achievement of the targets proposed by the Government and the World Health Organization.

Nurses expressed the conviction that primary health care opens new possibilities for research in the main areas of concern of the European strategy of Health for All: lifestyles and health; risk factors affecting health and environment; reorientation of health care systems and the political, managerial, technological, manpower and research support necessary to bring about the desired changes to achieve the targets. It was considered essential that the Government establish a national health research policy and set research priorities according to our own needs, with clear support to nursing research priorities.

Other important points concerning the future nursing research developments were identified by the nurses participating in the National Nursing Forum:

The need to develop a strategy for motivating universities, authorities, schools of nursing, health authorities at all levels – national, regional and local – as well as health care institutions to prepare nurse researchers and to conduct nursing research related to Health For All Targets.

Need for advanced nursing research training with emphasis on research designs and methodology, statistics and epidemiology, nursing theories and models, system analysis and operational research, economical and social sciences.

Need to promote changes in working conditions for nurse clinicians and university teachers doing research to provide them with enough time and adequate support for nursing research.

Need to develop a strategy to use the available financial resources in the Ministries of Health and Education, autonomic and local Governments, health institutions and private foundations.

Nurses need much more information on how to have access to available national and international funds and the possibility to present research projects to be funded by the European Economic Community or the Council of Europe Health Programs.

In summary, making the goal of Health for All by the Year 2000 a reality, depends particularly on facilitating the development of a body of knowledge which enhances nursing professional practice to achieve the delivery of appropriate care and better quality of nursing care for all the population.

It is also essential to recognize that development of nursing leadership is needed to support and increase nursing research.

## REFERENCES

Apilanez, V. (April 1983) 'Nurses' attitudes towards pain in cancer patients'. Unpublished research report presented at the First National Nursing Cancer Congress, Madrid.

General Council of Nursing (February 1988) *Research project to study the nursing situation in Spain*, Madrid.

Ministry of Education (July 1977) Royal Decree 922/1987. *Regulation of nursing specialties.* State Official Bulletin, Madrid.

Ministry of Education (May 1987) *Project for modification of directives for basic nursing education*, Ninth Commission Nursing Group, Council of Universities, Madrid.

Ministry of Health (1987) Royal Decree 521/1987. *Regulation of structure and organization of hospitals.* Official Bulletin.

Ministry of Health (December 1987) *Report on National Debates about Health for All Targets and Implications for the Nursing Profession*, Madrid.

Ovalle, M. (1984) *Interrelation of education practice and research, a strategy for development of primary health care.* Universidad Autonoma de Barcelona, Barcelona.

Ovalle, M. (1986) *Report on Development of Nursing Research in Spain.* 1983–1986. Meeting of Workgroup of European Nurse Researchers, Helsinki.

Ovalle, M. *et al.* (May 1988) *Survey on nursing continuing education*, General Council of Nursing, Madrid.

Report of the National Conference on Nursing and Primary Health care (Sponsored by Red Cross, University of Barcelona, Regional Government, WHO Regional Office for Europe, Geneva and WHO Geneva), Barcelona, 14–17 March 1983.

World Health Organization (1985) *Targets for Health for All: Targets in support of the European Regional Strategy for Health for All*, WHO, Regional Office for Europe, Copenhagen.

# CHAPTER SEVEN

# Primary health care nursing: development and research in Brazil

## Emilia Luigia Saporiti Angerami

This topic is first discussed on the basis of the situation in Latin America in general, followed by in-depth analysis of Brazil and of the specific aspects of its National Health System in which the nursing profession is inserted as it develops its practice, teaching and research functions. Projects that follow this integration model are presented at the end.

### THE LATIN-AMERICAN CONDITION

The efforts directed at transforming the health reality of less favoured populations, in view of the shocking disparity between developed countries and the so-called developing countries, find in the proposals of Primary Health Care (PHC) the concrete expression of the changes needed in the health policies of each nation, which to date have proved inadequate for the solution of the growing problems of this century.

We believe that for a better understanding of PHC in Brazil and of the involvement of nurses in this process it is necessary to go beyond frontiers and to look at these aspects within a wider historical, political, social and economic reality, i.e. the reality of Latin America. We recognize the diversity of Latin-American countries and the limitations of certain generalizations, but it is a fact that the common Iberian origin and three centuries of subordination to Spain and Portugal have left a legacy of similar sociopolitical problems and ideological and political behaviours in modern-day Latin-American countries.

According to Lambert (1969), from its initial formation to contemporary times, Latin America has historically evolved between backwardness and dependence, between generalized poverty and subordination, always under the weight of great losses. The historical condition of underdevelopment is seen by Galeano (1984) as dependence on the great centres of capitalism: 'From discovery to contemporary days, every feature was transformed into European, and later North American, capital and has been accumulating as such until today in distant centres of power. These features include the land, its fruits and its mineral-rich depths, the men and their working and consuming capacity, the natural resources and the human resources. The manner of production and the class structure of each place have been successively determined from the outside by being incorporated into the universal gears of capitalism.'

The political life of Latin America after independence has also known periods of repeated disturbances and instability marked by revolutions and authoritarian regimes – especially in the military form – with interruptions of the functioning of political and democratic institutions and aggravation of all existing imbalances and conflicts.

UNICEF (1987) data show that from 1980 to 1985 *per capita* income has fallen in 17 of the 23 countries in Latin America and that many of these countries are facing serious crises with their balance of payments. The foreign debt greatly exceeds the help, loans and export profits. In addition, considerable internal governmental spending has led the countries to unbearable deficits. UNICEF studies (1987) have concluded that in countries where the economic policy is determined by the International Monetary Fund, 'The standard of health and education services is declining in many countries and deteriorating health and nutrition is widespread among the young children of Africa and Latin America.' Another UNICEF report (1988) pointed out that, even though this is a very complex problem and a very difficult economic time, infant mortality around the world could be reduced from 38 000 per day (1987) to 33 000 or less by 1990 by proper education and transmission of information to the population.

Living in Latin America means accompanying the daily devastating effects of economic recession, with inflation reducing the purchasing power of thousands of people who live without housing or basic sanitation and are excluded from access to health and education services. The latter services are victims of the chronic inefficiency of the political and bureaucratic process, of the quantitative and qualitative deficiency of manpower and materials and of technological backwardness, since the deflationary policies set up by the various governments lead to a continuous reduction of funds for health and education.

The UNICEF report (1987), cited above, states that little is known about the repercussions of the present political and economic trends on the human dimension and questions the effects of such policies on mankind in general. We know that in addition to the population growth that occurred over the last decades, there were changes in the way of life: in 1950, 41% of the Latin-American population lived in urban areas; by 1980 the figure was 65% and the estimate of urban population growth for the year 2000 is 577% in relation to 1950 (OPAS/OMS, 1982b). The increased life expectancy in certain countries will be a matter of reflection about the growing numbers of the aged and the multiple factors involved in their care. This population will be relatively young and will continue to be exposed to the traditional health risks in addition to those faced by more socioeconomically developed countries.

Internal migration has created new social and health problems, especially in the large metropolitan centres, which are surrounded by peripheral zones of abject poverty, where unemployment, hunger and violence are associated with subhuman living, sanitation, health and education conditions.

In view of such a critical and uncertain situation which will probably last for some time, it seems opportune to point out the efforts that have been made in the health sector to face this tremendous challenge. After World War II, changes occurred in the economic and cultural dependence of Latin America, which shifted from an European to a North American colonizing emphasis. Thus, the text of the *Carta de Punta del Est*, part of the *Primeiro Plano Decenal das Nações Unidas para o Desenvolvimento*, is the juridical instrument for any type of continental action.

The Ten-year Plan of Public Health resulted from the inclusion of health, which became the norm for the 1962–71 programmes. From this initial plan, the concepts of the 1972–80 Ten-year Health Plan evolved, together with the joint declaration of the Health Departments of the Americas in 1977, which support the Primary Health Care project. Finally, in the Alma-Ata Declaration (1978), ratified by the World Health Assembly in 1979, Primary Care was adopted as a world strategy which will permit reaching the goal of 'Health for all by the Year 2000' (OPAS/OMS, 1973).

It was on the basis of this long search for 'social justice' in the Americas that the latest Action Plan was elaborated. The objective is as follows: 'More than any other single document the Action Plan represents a joint and solemn political commitment of the Governments who are members of this Organization to the peoples of the Americas in order to reach a level of health that will permit each individual in this Region to lead a socially and economically productive life (OPAS/OMS, 1982a).

Health professionals reading this document will learn about governmental directives, about the kind of commitment they should make in practice, and which goals are to be reached. Marginal populations, children, women in the childbearing years, the elderly and the handicapped have the highest priority. The Action Plan suggests how the health delivery systems could operate and be reformulated, becoming more efficient and effective and responding to the effect of the policies and projects of economic development on health and on the population, with ties established among the various sectors.

The focal point of our work is Primary Health Care, which, according to the definition approved at Alma-Ata, is something more than limited, primary level care based on simple technology for marginal populations. Rather, it is a transformation of the entire health system in a given society.

## BRAZIL – A LATIN-AMERICAN UNIT

Brazil is the largest country in Latin America, covering eight and a half million square kilometres, which corresponds to approximately 40% of the total area of the South American continent.

Despite its position in South America, Brazil is viewed by Ribeiro (1979) as a socially and economically separate unit, since the vast extension of its borders separates it from its neighbouring countries rather than providing access to them because of the precarious means of land communication and the immense uninhabited areas in its territory. However, possible integration factors may be pointed out if we consider that the Brazilian people have become aware of the exploitation by North America and have therefore been forced to progress in a continental effort aimed at economic parity through a mutually satisfactory common market.

The Brazilian people are multicultural and multiracial, with the most important contributions coming from Indians, Blacks and Europeans. In 1980, the population of Brazil reached 119 070 865 people, corresponding to 30% of the entire population of the Latin-American continent (IBGE, 1982). The ethnic composition of Brazil is characterized by miscegenation of the various ethnic groups with each other and with the Portuguese in particular, who, in the process of domination, imposed their language, their religion and a social order favouring their own interests. These differences, however, were amalgamated into a vigorous national self-definition, which, according to Ribeiro (1979), has become increasingly Brazilian and has been a source of encouragement to the people.

The profound differences that separate the Brazilians are the blatantly contrasting strata at the social level. The privileged circles that were able to reach high standards of consumerism in the midst of a generally penurious economy are distinct from the enormous mass that lives at the margin of the productive process and of the cultural, social and political life of the nation.

The age composition of the Brazilian population, as estimated in 1980, is as follows: 37.4% less than 15 years; 58.3% 15–64 years, and 4.3% 65 years and older (IBGE, 1982). It can be seen that the population is predominantly young, representing high costs in the health and education areas with no immediate returns, because this is still an economically inactive population.

The worldwide demographic explosion that has occurred since 1950, especially in underdeveloped countries, is due to multiple causes. All of them, however, basically result from a major factor, i.e. the poverty in which millions of human beings live (Adas, 1982). As the author comments, 'the reduction in the mortality rate that occurred in Latin America after 1940–50 was not accompanied by a similar reduction in birth rate'. A recent study on the birth rate in Brazil, however, has reported a 25% drop from 1965 to 1975, including the depressed north-east (Draibe *et al.*, 1986).

The territorial space belonging to the Brazilian population today is the consequence of a faulty historical leadership and economic situation, whereby the established land-ownership structure prevents better exploitation of the land, with increasing tensions in this area. The urban space also represents a point of conflict, since the rural exodus and the internal migrations have caused the agglomeration of vast population contingents near the large cities, with consequent serious problems in terms of quality of life due to the inability of the urban space to absorb the disorderly population growth.

Still considering space distribution, I would like to emphasize the role of industrialization. Brazil is one of the most dynamic and diversified countries in this sector, with most of its industrial area located in the south-east, where the State of São Paulo is the major industrial centre accounting for 56.7% of the total Brazilian national product. This strong industrial concentration generates imbalances, such as that existing between the south-east and the north-east. The south-eastern region attracts and polarizes human and material resources because of its key position on the national scene, whereas the north-east has fewer economic and social resources, resulting in a marked retardation of development as compared with the rest of the country.

This disparity, though not so marked, also exists in relation to the south and centre-west regions, in which production is centred on ore exploitation, cattle-raising and agriculture, which are very important factors in the economic life of the country.

Because of its geographic location, the Amazon region (north) represents a peculiar question with respect to national integration.

These regional differences stem from geographic, climatic, socio-economic and cultural factors, which markedly affect the health of the population and the delivery of services. Recognizing these regional differences is of fundamental importance for the understanding of the health-sickness and education processes, since they have different characteristics in each subregion and require the health system to adapt in terms of manpower, technology and politics.

## NATIONAL HEALTH POLICY

Brazil has reached one of its more remarkable political moments, i.e. democratic transition after twenty years of military dictatorship. The focal point of the political process is the elaboration of a new Constitution which will determine a new sociopolitical order. This political moment, taken together with the economic pressures that burden the country, is the background for the health reform which formulates the legal basis for the health system.

The structure of the health sector always followed the changes that occurred in the socioeconomic structure. Born at the beginning of the century within the capitalist coffee economy, the structure mainly involved questions of urban and port sanitation. During the economic crisis of the twenties and the incipient process of industrialization, the emphasis shifted to the individual: because of the need for manpower and productivity, the social welfare system was introduced around 1930 in order to protect workers, with the creation of the so-called 'Institutes'. These 'Institutes' were founded by professional bodies, but successive transformations led to the creation in 1967 of a single organ represented by the National Welfare and Social Assistance Institute. Over the years the Institute extended coverage to 23% of the population (1966) and to 87% by 1983, representing perhaps the largest welfare system in the world (Jouval, 1985).

Medical companies and private hospitals blossomed during the 1960s, a phenomenon that should be understood in the light of the industrialization process, which gained new impetus in the late 1950s. At that time the relationship between State and Capital was so strong that it made its mark on health. The government took on the responsibility of offering assistance to all workers and, since the public service network was not equipped for this, the services of private clinics were bought. Several assistance plans were developed along this model, but were not successful.

At the end of the 1970s, the disorganization of government activities was widely known and the need was felt to rationalize both the activities and costs of hospital units, which had been growing alarmingly. During the present decade, attempts have been made to reverse this process at different levels of coverage and complexity. At the technical level, particularly noteworthy was the approval, in August 1983, of the 'Plan of Reorientation of Health Care within the Area of Social Welfare', which gave priority to primary health care and to the integration of government-supported health institutions (at the federal, state and local level) into a single regionalized and hierarchic service. This plan, which was implemented in 1983 and was maintained until 1984, was followed by a new strategy called Integrated Health Actions (IHA).

The IHA programme is based on the assumption that the control of the health system and the health of the population are the full responsibility of the political power. It also assumes the integration of institutions, health planning, actions preventing preventive/curative, individual/collective, ambulatory/hospital dichotomies. It is still too early for an evaluation.

However, according to Draibe *et al.* (1986) the perspective is that the measures taken thus far will result in increased coverage, rationalization of costs and technological recovery and adequacy through integration with the agencies that finance science and technology.

In the field of human resources there was a reduction of salary disparities and a stimulation of training of middle-level professionals.

The areas of the programme which have been given priority by the Health Departments are:

Medical-Sanitary Assistance

Control of Transmissible diseases

Sanitary Control

Infrastructure for basic heath and sanitation services and institutional
    development.

Two political moments have given continuity to this process of revision of the health sector: the Eighth National Health Conference of 1986, and the Health Reform Implantation project, which is currently under way in the country.

As pointed out earlier, the regional differences of Brazil affect the entire process, since even when a plan has a national character, the different health realities, human and technological resources and socioeconomic characteristics at the regional level require all kinds of adjustments.

In 1980, 180 048 children less than 1 year old died in Brazil, and in the same year 24 in 100 deaths occurred in this age group, showing the importance of this problem. Infant mortality was 85.2 per one thousand live births in 1977, with the following regional differences: north, 76.9, north-east, 99.0; and south-east, 92.5, the highest rates; centre-west, 85.2, and south, 68.6, the lowest rate. The predominant causes of death are enteritis, pneumonia and other perinatal causes (Yunes, Campos and Carvalho, 1987). In the poorest regions (north–north-east), the primary cause of death is still represented by infectious and parasitic diseases, followed by circulatory disease, whereas the latter takes first place in the more advanced centres.

## INVOLVEMENT OF NURSING IN THE HEALTH SYSTEM

Nursing practice in Latin America has been analysed in depth by Verderese (1980) in relation to health practices and the socioeconomic structure. The study defines nursing practice accompanying the development of current health models and characterizes it as always directed towards hospital care, i.e., as more of a curative than a preventive type of practice. The changes that took place during the last two decades in the philosophy and methods of care have had repercussions on nursing, provoking criticism of its practice and teaching. Thus, several programmes arose involving an extension of coverage, a revision of curricular structure and a concern with the development of greater integration between teaching and service.

The accepted notion that auxiliary staff and community agents play an important role in primary care programs required a revision of the nurse's role, which appears to be one of co-ordination and leadership in health practice. However, even though this was the proposal, Chompré *et al.* (1986), in a survey carried out in Latin America, observed that no nurses at the IHA level had been contracted by any of the services. As to the health system, the authors observed that in all the countries that they visited attempts were being made to extend coverage through the organization of primary care services, but the coexistence of this practice with the growing privatization of medicine is making the organization of this first level quite difficult. They described the teaching of nursing as still traditional, with a gap between teaching and practice. As to the latter, the major obstacle for good performance is the level of competence and specialization.

In Brazil, 304 287 people are currently engaged in nursing practice, and are distributed as follows: nurses 8.5%; practical nurses 6.6%; nurses's aides 21.1%, and attendants 63.8% (Brazil/Cofen, 1985). It should be emphasized that this distribution, which represents the profile of the country, is not the same for all geographical regions, since there are states in which the percentage of nurses is much lower and the percentage of attendants much higher. According to the same report, the nursing labour force is mostly distributed between hospitals (70.4%) and public health services (27.9%). The remaining 1.4% work in teaching institutions and perform other activities such as work in independent clinics.

In addition to representing an evaluation of national priorities in the question of training of manpower both in qualitative and quantitative terms, these data show how many of the problems related to teaching, practice and research have multiple causes and require profound structural changes. As an example, I shall mention a change in salary policy, expansion of job opportunities, appreciation of nursing work, and definition of the nurse's role in the health sector.

Ideologically, nurses have been 'called' to take their place in the health team and in this respect, Angerami and Almeida (1983), in a discussion of the nurse's role, have warned about the need to eliminate repetitive practice in order to transform reality through a creative praxis.

Efforts have been made over the last two decades to develop research and to systematize knowledge, which is mainly generated by graduate courses. This production, however, is still not expressed at the national level when compared to other areas of health knowledge in general. This production also has regional characteristics, i.e., it is concentrated in the south-east, which is the most developed region in the country.

The Nursing Study and Research Centre (CEPEn) has stimulated reflection among nurses by promoting several investigation seminars which have given them an opportunity to discuss their 'praxis' and the relationship with the production of knowledge. Methodological questions have also been studied in depth in an attempt to understand that the construction of knowledge is a slow and complementary process and that the most important aspect is the quality and social significance attributed to it. It is from this focal point of view that I would like to approach the considerations that follow, which originate from the questions: Why do we carry out research? Who are the recipients of our research? Research should permeate teaching and practice and, in this respect, I would like to go back to the background described in the earlier part of this chapter.

In most Latin-American countries, in which the sharp disparity between social classes has not yet been eliminated, the health systems are based on the privilege of certain groups who enjoy highly sophisticated services, while a large portion of the population has no access to the minimal health and environmental conditions that are needed for survival. A bureaucratic model prevails in health centres, with rigidly set rules and regulations, whereby a person, with his/her inalienable right to health, has no say and is subjected to the power plays that permeate the entire system.

Nursing is included in the system with the characteristic of the so-called team, not in the philosophical meaning of the term but because it consists of at least three categories with different training, which, however, play the same roles and execute the same functions while receiving debasing salaries for their work.

The nurse, pressed by the bureaucratization of services and by the hegemony of doctors, tries to establish her position in her practice, but when the objective of her work – patient care – is sought an army of attendants is faced, carrying out tasks for which they received in-service training.

This is the reality of our praxis. Research, whose starting and end points are based on praxis, should contribute to the identification of problems and the search for solutions. This emerging praxis should be critical, capable of overcoming the classic dichotomy between knowing and doing and able to generate actions that will permit the free exercise of the profession.

If, on the one hand, nursing research in Brazil could be considered as still limited, it should be pointed out that it has been progressively growing and that it has contributed to the revelation and explanation of some phenomena. The aim of our efforts, however, is to be able to reach and transform nursing practice through the knowledge produced.

The path pointed out for transforming praxis is based on the primary care model, which could reduce the existing disparities. On this basis, I looked for studies planned and developed by nurses which focused on primary health care, on national priorities such as the health of women, children and workers, and were carried out in collaboration with service professionals while at the same time proposing investigation and teaching. My criterion for the selection of these studies was based on personal acquaintance and exchange with the researchers, a fact that facilitated the task considerably.

The Breast-feeding Nucleus ('Núcleo de Aleitamento Materno', NALMA) of the Nursing School of Ribeirão Preto was created during the present decade on the basis of the cumulative experience of a group of nurses engaged in assistance to the mother–child relationship in an attempt to promote breast-feeding. Because of its broad scope and performance, it is considered a national centre for the training of health professionals. The activities of the centre include teaching, research and service in the hospital, outpatient clinic and community. The centre is staffed by members of the Nursing School faculty, nurses, doctors, undergraduate and graduate students and trainees.

By helping mothers through the lactation period, NALMA attempts to develop maternal identity based on the model of Rubin (1985) and the self-care concept of Orem (1985), with strong emphasis on educational support. In terms of research, the focal point is the appropriate technology for self-care with respect to the post partum breast using the mother's hand and the baby's suction for milk expression (Shimo, Vinha and Ferreira, 1985; Vinha *et al.*, 1985; Vinha, 1987). After NALMA was set up, the incidence of weaning due to mammary factors among the treated population fell to zero (Vinha, 1988). The procedures adopted for the prophylaxis and treatment of breast engorgement, mammillary trauma and mastitis were applicable and useful for the mothers, who showed competence and ease in following them.

The inclusion of nurses of the Nursing School of Ribeirão Preto in School Health started in 1981 with a pilot project from which resulted the Primary School Health Care Programme (PROASE). PROASE, which today has agreements with government bodies and is integrated in the national health policy, utilizes the teaching-assistance strategy in order to promote man and to help him understand his own reality more deeply. The work is focused on children and aims at remedying the socioeconomic problems that affect school and education in an attempt to transform these two very complex realities.

Doctors, nurses, dentists, psychologists, teachers, university professors and students of the different professions participate in a multiprofessional team providing care to 6146 children at six schools in a peripheral area of the city. Decentralization, use of appropriate technology, participation of auxiliary personnel and interinstitutional integration in a system of referral with existing teams at primary health stations are the main characteristics of PROASE activity.

The nurse carries out educational, supportive and administrative functions and plays a relevant political role with respect to the agencies participating in the agreement (Ferriani, 1988). This author reports that in an assessment carried out in 1986, the nurse's work reached a high level of problem solving in terms of basic actions, with a perceptible reduction in referrals. The most frequent conditions were accidents, parasitic diseases, and hearing, visual and respiratory problems. The author also discusses the high percentage of repeaters during the first years of school and the psychosocial difficulties that permeate the lives of these children.

It is the intention of the State Secretariat to start immediate use of this model which originated from the integration of a researcher into the daily life of schoolchildren in an administrative area that covers 22 cities in the State of São Paulo.

The Trans-sector Community Action Programme (PTAC), developed by the Federal University of Minas Gerais and by institutions providing primary health care to rural and peripheral communities through a multi-professional team consisting of teachers and students, is based on teaching-assistance integration aimed at training professionals who are aware of the reality of these communities and who participate in the service-providing institutions (Costa *et al.* 1985).

The nursing school plays a leading role in this process which was first set up in 1985. Even though research is not yet a primary component of this process, it can be seen that, as the teaching practice of the school at the basic service level becomes broader and more systematized, the essential foundations for teaching, research and extension are consolidated (Araujo and Chompré, 1986).

The teaching/assistance experience has led the school to question the Nursing curriculum and the teaching of Nursing as a whole, with consequent rethinking of the training of nurses and other nursing workers. Internship in rural zones has been playing a decisive role for the qualitative and quantitative redefinition of nurses engaged in basic health care, leading the organizations involved to include nurses in health centres. The studies carried out thus far have permitted the accumulation of some knowledge, with a decrease in the gap existing in the primary health area. A project for the development of nursing in Latin-America was elaborated in 1987 with the objective of improving graduate courses involving primary care with the support of the W.K. Kellogg Foundation.

## CONCLUSION

The preceding exposition is an attempt to show that the concept of PHC should ge beyond the limits of a discussion of the theoretical/practical model of assistance and to grasp the sociopolitical meaning of PHC as a transformer of health systems.

The divergences between society and State are a permanent challenge in Latin America. Thus, it will only be through the application of nurses and of all other health workers to the political struggle currently under way in health systems that the possibility of transforming established and anachronistic structures into dynamic services freely accessible to the entire population may turn into a reality.

The articulation of teaching, research and practice has been a constant goal even though the desired success has not yet been obtained. Appropriation of knowledge occurs in teaching, but knowledge cannot be appropriated unless its theoretical dimension is understood. Thus, it is in the search for this theoretical foundation that the health professional will occupy his/her full position and be able to practice the critical reflection needed to understand the educational process and its proper praxis. This praxis has proved to be alienated, non-creative, repetitive and boring, since workers are forbidden to produce knowledge.

The dividing line between those who think and investigate and those who apply knowledge in practice has obstructed the advances needed to solve problems involved in providing services. For this reason it is important for the University to look for political channels leading to the community and to be engaged in a participating manner so as to disperse doubts about its decisive role in the process of change.

The examples presented above reveal that, in addition to political engagement, a teaching/assistance involvement and a commitment to team work has occurred, favouring the participation of all concerned.

Praxis based on a critical vision of social reality is an ample source of questions to be studied. Furthermore, it represents a manner of providing health care with health objectives directed at the real needs of the population and based on competent knowledge that will contribute to a better quality of life and to the construction of a more just society.

## REFERENCES

Adas, M. (1982) *Geografia da América: Aspectos da Geografia Fisica e Social*, Editora Moderna, São Paulo.

Alma-Ata (1978) *Conferencia Internacional Sobre Atención Primaria de Salud, 6–12 de Septiembre de 1978.* Organización Mundial de la Salud/Fondo de las Naciones Unidas para la Infancia (Serie 'Salud para todos', no. 1). Ginebra-Nueva York.

Angerami, E.L.S. and Almeida, M.C.P. (1983) De como o enfermeiro está inserido no seu espaço, *Educación Médica y Salud,* **17**, 150–163, PAHO/WHO, Washington.

Araujo, M.R.N. de and Chompré, R.R. (1986) Relato de la Experiencia de Integración Docente Asistencial de la Escuela de Enfermeria de la Universidad Federal de Minas Gerais (UFMG). *La Enfermeria en Latino América. Estrategias para su desarrollo. Memorias de la reunión de lideranzas de enfermeria. Caracas, marzo, 1985. Federación Panamericana e Asociaciones de Facultades e Escuelas de Medicina (FEPAC).* Caracas, Venezuela (Publicación no. 8, 57–71).

Brazil/COFEN (1985). *O Exercicio da Enfermagem nas Instituições de Saúde do Brasil: 1982/1983*. Força de trabalho em enfermagem, vol. I. Conselho Federal de Enfermagem/Associação Brasileira de Enfermagem, Rio de Janeiro.

Chompré, R.R. *et al.* (co-ordinators) (1986) *Seminário de Viagens de Enfermeiras Docentes-assistenciais que Atuam em Programas de Assistência Primária. Relatório 1986*. Centro Audiovisual/Universidade Federal de Minas Gerais, Belo Horizonte.

Costa, A.E., Corrêa, E.J., Chompré, R.R. *et al.* (1985) Programa transetorial de ação comunitária, Aspectos preliminares de seu desenvolvimento. *REDES*, Lima (Peru) no. 5: 22–27.

Draibe, S.M. *et al.* (co-ordinators) (1986) *Brasil 1985: Relatório Sobre a Situação Social do Pais*. Núcleo de Estudos em Politicas Públicas – Instituto de Economia da UNICAMP, vol. I, Campinas.

Ferriani, M.G. (1988) *A Inserção do Enfermeiro na Saúde Escolar – Análise Critica de Uma Experiência*, unpublished Doctoral thesis, Nursing School of Ribeirão Preto.

Galeano, E. (1984) *As Veias Abertas da América Latina* (translated by Galeno de Freitas), 19th edn, Editora Paz e Terra, Rio de Janeiro (Collection 'Estudos Latino-Americanos', vol. 12).

IBGE (1982) *Anuário Estatistico do Brasil*. Fundação Instituto Brasileiro de Geografia e Estatistica, vol 43, Rio de Janeiro.

Jouval, H. (1985) A integração de sistemas de assistência primária à saúde. Tema I. *Medicina*, **18**, 8–36.

Lambert, J. (1969) *América latina: estruturas sociais e instituições politicas*, Editora Nacional e Editora da USP, São Paulo.

OPAS/OMS (1973) *Plan decenal de salud para las Américas. Informe final de la III Reunión Especial de Ministros de Salud de las Américas (Santiago, Chile. 2–9 de octubre de 1972)*. Documento Oficial no. 118, Organización Panamericana de la Salud/Organización Mundial de la Salud, Washington.

OPAS/OMS (1982a) *Salud para todos en el año 2,000: plan de acción para la instrumentación de las estrategias regionales*. Documento Oficial no. 179, Organización Panamericana de la Salud/Organización Mundial de la Salud, Washington.

OPAS/OMS (1982b) *Las condiciones de salud en las Américas 1977–1980*. Publicación Cientifica no. 427, Organización Panamericana de la Salud/ Organización Mundial de la Salud, Washington.

Orem, E.D. (1985) *Nursing Concepts of Practice*, 3rd edn, McGraw-Hill, New York.

Ribeiro, D. (1979) *As Américas e a civilização: estudos de antropologia da civilização*. Editora Vozes Ltda., Petropolis.

Rubin, R. (1985) *Maternal Identity and the Maternal Experience*, Springer, New York.

Shimo, A.K.K., Vinha, V.H.P. and Ferreira, D.L.B. (1985) Mama puerperal: uma proposta de cuidados. *Femina*, **13**, 159–166.

UNICEF (1987) *The State of the World's Children*. United Nations Children's Fund, Oxford University Press, Oxford.

UNICEF (1988) *Situação mundial da infância*. Fundo das Nações Unidas para a Infância, Brasilia.

Verderese, O. (1980) Análisis de la enfermeria en la América Latina. *Antologia de experiencias en servicio y docencia en enfermeria en América.* Publicación Cientifica no. 393, 1–17, OPAS/OMS, Washington.

Vinha, V.H.P. (1987) *Amamentação Materna: Incentivo e Cuidados,* 2a. edn, Sarvier, São Paulo.

Vinha, V.H.P. (1988) *Projeto aleitamento materno:determinação de sua eficácia com vistas ao auto-cuidado com a mama puerperal.* Unpublished 'Livre Docência' thesis, Nursing School of Ribeirão Preto.

Vinha, V.H.P., Pelá, N.T.R., Shimo, A.K.K. *et al.* (1985) Trauma mamilar: avaliação de uma proposta de tratamento. *Femina,* **15**, 370–378.

Yunes, J., Campos, O. and Carvalho, V.S.S. (1987) Assistência à infância, à adolescência e a maternidade no Brasil. *Boletin de la Oficina Sanitaria Pan-americana,* **103**, 33–42, OPAS/OMS, Washington.

# CHAPTER EIGHT

# Chronicity research over the life cycle in Israel

*Miriam J. Hirschfeld and Tamar Krulik*

## INTRODUCTION

Israel, celebrating the 40th anniversary of independence this year, is a small country between Europe and Asia on the Eastern Coast of the Mediterranean. The population is composed of 3.3 million Jews and 640 000 Arabs.

Within less than a generation the demographic and morbidity patterns in Israel changed from those of a developing to those of a developed country. For example, while in the early 1950s infectious diseases were the major causes of morbidity for the entire population, today cardiovascular and cerebrovascular diseases, cancer and stress-related syndromes are the major healthcare problems for all. In the Jewish population the proportion of elderly has risen from 3.7% in 1950 to 10% in 1988.

The developed countries of the world had the entire century to adapt their health care services from a focus on infectious diseases and acute care to services which could meet the needs of chronicity and long-term care. The developing countries, on the other hand, are faced with providing these same services while also dealing with other overwhelmingly competing demands, such as population control and the coverage of basic needs (e.g. food and housing). Israel's unique development provides a paradigm case example on which to demonstrate the effects of rapid demographic, economic, social and morbidity changes reflected in the health care system.

Israel has attempted to meet health care challenges through a basic commitment to provide health care services to all its citizens. General health care services developed over a period of thirty years preceding the establishment of the State set a solid foundation for today's comprehensive health care in the country. However, although the services have reached remarkable standards, today the general (public) health care system is in jeopardy.

## THE ISRAELI HEALTH CARE SYSTEM

Ninety-six per cent of Israel's population is insured by one of the four sick funds which cover health care services in the public sector. The remaining 4% have sufficient income to meet their health care expenditures. Kupat Holim, the sick fund of the General Federation of Labor insures close to 80% of the population, which includes special coverage for the poor paid for by the Ministry of Health and provides the majority of primary care in some 1300 community clinics in both urban and rural areas. The Ministry of Health maintains maternal and child stations with overall responsibility for preventive care. Services to healthy mothers and children are well developed. However, services to chronically ill or disabled children and their families lag behind the need. While community-based preventive and long-term care is developing at a steady pace, long-term care services are still insufficient to meet the rapidly growing needs of all age groups.

Payment of hospitalization is covered by the sick funds and is provided in public hospitals (Ministry of Health, Kupat Holim and Hadassah) to the entire population. Recently, as a result of prolonged budgetary and labour relation crisis in the public sector (strikes of all sectors including two prolonged physician strikes and a nurses' hunger strike), private hospitals and community services have expanded and threaten the integrity of the public system. Long-term institutional care is provided by both the public and private sectors, but availability of affordable, quality care services continues to be a major problem.

The traditional ideology of an egalitarian health care system was the basis for the development of the comprehensive public health service. However, rapidly rising health care costs, increasing demands and expectations coupled with a waning social commitment to 'Health for All', create strains on the public health system and jeopardize its viability.

## MAJOR NURSING PROBLEMS

The worldwide health care crisis has impacted nursing internationally, and the nursing problems of Israel are remarkably similar to those found in many other parts of the world (Aiken and Mullinex, 1987; Delamothe, 1988; Dunea, 1988). In Israel today nursing is in a state of crisis, characterized by an acute awareness of the gap between the growing demands upon the profession and the inability to meet these demands under the present circumstances. This is especially so, since because of higher education and a growing body of nursing research, nurses know that they have a vital service to offer. Nurses are deeply troubled, as they realize that the present health care climate threatens not only the provision of vital services, but the further development of nursing education and research.

The last decade of fiscal crisis resulted in cuts of nursing positions and in nurses electing to move from full- to part-time positions. In the same period the patient population, older, sicker and far more dependent, demanded more nursing care. This unprecedented burden and the inability to adequately respond to care needs, combined with inadequate pay and working conditions, have led nurses to leave the public sector and seek employment in private facilities. Those who stay in the public health care system and who care for the vast majority of the population feel even more frustrated, exploited and burdened. Along with these changes, strikes and unfavourable coverage by the media have led to a further erosion in the image of the nursing profession.

This situation threatens to erode the great strides made in nursing education and research over the last decades. There are now high-level academic programmes for nursing in three major universities in addition to non-degree nursing education programmes. Graduates are well regarded in service and they develop research and quality care. The present major problem is a decreasing number of applicants to schools of nursing. The decline in new graduates, in nursing students and in applicants has reached an alarming level and adds to the feeling of burden, since nurses do not foresee positive developments in the near future. Nursing finds itself in a vicious circle of a growing demand for 'working hands' and fewer qualified nurses now and in the future willing and able to answer the need. The fact that nurses know that, with different priorities in resource allocation (more nursing positions, better pay and improved working conditions) this trend could be reversed, makes the situation more difficult to tolerate.

As mentioned above, Israel today has health care and nursing problems similar to those of most of the developed world. As a result, there are a plethora of unanswered questions in need of research. The following sections address the efforts of Israeli nurses to develop part of this body of knowledge.

## NURSING RESEARCH – THE STATE OF THE ART

In the past research was conducted primarily in academic settings by faculty or students completing their higher degrees. In the past decade various agencies and practising nurses have also become involved in research activities. The Israeli Nursing Association recently established a committee for nursing research with the hope that the association will take a major role in encouraging and facilitating nursing research. In addition, in several large medical centres positions were allocated for nurses to establish and initiate nursing research.

The research generated by these positions usually includes participation by groups of hospital nurses, who use the survey method to focus on such issues as accidents, errors in medication and falls among the elderly.

Principles of nursing research have been included in all baccalaureate nursing curricula. In addition, some students take part in advanced research seminars and perform group research. All masters students must complete an original thesis as part of the degree requirement. Nurses in practice are learning about research findings in evening lectures and study days presented by university faculty, as well as in biennial conferences, in which many papers are research based. These lectures and conferences stimulate nurses to implement research findings to change practice. The nursing leadership has been able to attract international conferences to Israel, so that Israeli nurses can present their own research and hear about research being done by others.

In an effort to categorize our work, the first inventory of nursing research in Israel was published in 1970 by the Department of Nursing, Tel Aviv University. It included 30 items whereas the last inventory, published in 1987, reported on 182 studies. The increase indicates the growing interest and expertise of nurses in research, as well as the readiness of agencies to initiate and/or support such efforts (Bergman, 1987).

Research completed to date represents the following areas: (1) nursing history, (2) clinical nursing, (3) nursing administration including manpower, (4) nursing education, and (5) social and anthropological aspects of health and illness.

We have to date been involved primarily in survey and descriptive studies. but see increasing emphasis on interventional studies. We are also ready to forge linkages in our research efforts. First, in our own country we will begin to link individual nursing studies into groups and centres across the country. At the same time, we will encourage linkages to our colleagues in other disciplines. And, finally, we will increase our present efforts to link with international colleagues to develop more cross-cultural studies.

With these efforts we can expect nursing research in Israel to continue to grow and develop, and add to the ever-increasing internationally-generated body of nursing knowledge.

The following is an example of our internal linkage of individual interest to form common studies.

## RESEARCH ON DEPENDENCY CARE AND THE FAMILY

With changing demographic and morbidity patterns chronicity and dependency care have become a major challenge for nursing. Before describing some of the specific Israeli research in this area we shall focus on the conceptualization guiding this research development. Research in many countries attests the well-known fact that the major responsibility for dependency care is with the family. We, therefore, perceive 'the family' as the focus of research, both in its ability to give care to dependent family members, as well as in its need for attention and care from nursing as a group at risk in need of guidance and support.

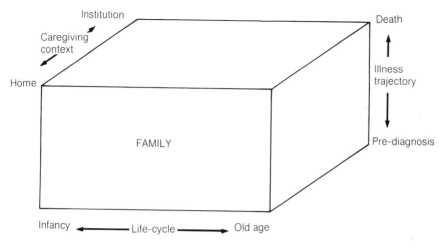

**Figure 8.1** 'The family' as the focus of research.

Research is looking at the phenomenon of family caregiving as related to: (1) the kind of impairment, (2) the point along the life-cycle, and (3) the illness trajectory-place context of home to institutional care.

1. *Impairment* This aspect is based on the non-categorical approach (Stein and Jessop, 1982), which does not see the essential differences in caregiving related to the medical diagnoses, but the kind of impairment and handicap. Cardinal questions from this vantage point are the difficulties faced by the family when dealing with physical versus mental impairment; or management strategies with medical versus behavioural symptoms and their social consequences.

2. *Life-cycle* This research aspect is concerned with the aspects related to growth and development of those who receive and give family care alike. 'Patients' in family care can be, for instance, infants with birth defects, school-age children who are dying, adolescents who have psychotic conditions, young mothers or fathers with malignant or degenerative diseases, or an old person who is bedridden or senile. Caregivers are young parents to their children, spouses of all ages – from the very young to the very old – (old women are today the main group of caregivers to the aged), – middle-aged children to the old; but also children give care to their chronically ill, handicapped or dying siblings or parents. Factors related to the growth and development of the patient, the caregiver and the family as an entity in itself, are all crucial variables, which must be understood in family care.

3. The caregiving context addresses questions related to when and where care is given. Caregiving before and around diagnosis is different from that given during periods of maintenance or remission, exacerbation of

disease, or during the final stage. There are different problems to face when giving care in the home or in the institution and different questions involved in deciding upon the feasibility of home care at the start, or moving from home to institutional care. Family involvement and abdication of care interlink with questions related to social and health care policy and general social values.

A major research project on this area in Israel is 'Family care for the severely handicapped children and aged in Israel' (Krulik, Hirschfeld and Sharon, 1984).

There is a growing number of children and aged with severe chronic health problems in the community. Mothers become the prime caregivers to these children; ageing spouses or middle-aged offspring are the caregivers to these aged. In-depth interviews were conducted with 92 families of impaired children and 181 families of impaired aged in their homes.

The research describes caregivers who in the face of tremendous hardship wish to continue home care to their severely impaired children and adult relatives. Several major findings arose from this study:

1. In contrast to what might be expected from social stereotypes there was little difference between caregivers to children or to elderly in regard to their readiness and ability to undertake home care, once they have opted to care for an impaired relative;
2. Most caregivers perceived caregiving to have some negative effect upon one or more of three major areas in their lives:
   (a) Physical and mental health;
   (b) The caregiver's daily basic needs such as privacy, a sense of security, the opportunity to leave the house and the ability for rest and work;
   (c) Family and social relationships;
3. The variation of caregivers' perception of the overall burden was not related to demographic variables such as sex, age, educational level, country of origin and level of religious observance. It was also unrelated to the functional ability (ADL) of patients, or to the caregiving duration or intensity. However, the perception of burden was related to the kind of impairment and the caregiving trajectory for caregivers of adults. Burden was highest when the patient suffered from mental impairment only and lowest where there was only physical impairment. The more the caregiver perceived the situation to be growing worse, the greater she/he perceived the overall cost;
4. The variation of caregivers' tolerance and management ability of symptoms/behaviour was related to several variables. For the child population the symptoms which posed the greatest difficulty were faecal incontinence, sleep disturbance and impaired communication. Among the ageing patients falls and instability, faecal incontinence,

impaired communication and sleep disturbance were the most difficult to manage. Carers found that among the sick children dangerous, aggressive, violent, uncooperative and restless behaviour were the most difficult to tolerate and manage, while among the aged patients dangerous, uncooperative and apathetic behaviours posed the greatest difficulties;

5. The majority of caregivers to both populations rejected institutionalization as a viable option;

   The variation of caregivers' attitudes toward institutionalization was related to several variables. Caregivers, who were willing to consider institutionalization as a potential alternative to home-care were:

   (a) Mothers who had a number of small children and those who had a lower level of formal education and less economic resources. Demographic variables made no difference for the caregivers to adults;

   (b) Caregivers who perceived their patient to be deteriorating;

   (c) Caregivers who felt that their physical health was negatively affected by caregiving;

   (d) Those who considered themselves depressed and anxious;

6. The quality of the caregiver–patient relationship and the perceived gratitude of patients in both populations were crucial for a positive outlook toward continuation of home care.

Three research projects highlighting different aspects on family care of the aged followed the above work.

Two studies focused on specific aspects of home care and one study addressed what happens to caregivers when home care breaks down.

Lindenbaum (1989) developed a tool to study the caregiver–patient relationship. This variable arose as the crucial factor in the family intent to continue home care in prior research (Hirschfeld, 1983; Krulik, Hirschfeld and Sharon, 1984). In this research the Attachment theory (Bowlby, 1982) served as the conceptual frame underlying the tool construction. This tool measures attachment in a caregiving situation and Lindenbaum demonstrated, again, that this variable is crucial for caregiving spouses to tolerate and continue home care. Her sample included 71 spouses (45 wives and 26 husbands) caring for severely demented patients, who she interviewed at their homes. These caregivers felt great pride in their ability to master a most difficult situation. The greater the caregiving burden, the greater seemed their satisfaction and attachment. This indicates that the successful mastery of a most difficult challenge is possibly a powerful motivator for those families, who choose to continue such difficult home care.

In an additional project Hirschfeld *et al.* (unpublished) constructed a tool to measure the frequency and intensity of symptoms and patient or family ability to tolerate and cope with symptoms or behaviours. Successful symptom control is an aspect of family caregiving crucial to the well-being of patients and caregivers alike.

Gerstanski (1986) explored the effect of institutionalization upon families. She interviewed 60 caregivers, who had cared for their demented family members from two to 19 years at home. Institutionalization was a last resort. The main question of this study was to what extent institutionalization had brought physical and emotional relief to the family caregiver. Twenty-two family caregivers were spouses and 38 were children of demented patients.

The main findings were that most caregivers felt relief after institutionalizing their demented relatives as compared to the time when they had cared for them at home. With that, approximately one-fourth felt guilty, helpless, restless, lonely and unable to utilize their newly-gained free time.

This leads to the conclusion, that the two main factors determining the impact of institutionalization are the family caregivers' ability to overcome separation from the patient, as well as their resources to rebuild their own life.

Bergman and Gerstanski (1987) add to our understanding of the phenomenon of family caregiving within the institution. The aim of their study was to develop an instrument to examine the quality of care of patients in psychogeriatric units. They gathered data from interviews with patients, staff and families (N = 33) and conducted participant observations on six psychogeriatric units. In relation to family caregiving they arrived at the following conclusions: families play a major role in the quality of care of patients, also in the institution; they differ in their wish to be involved with direct patient care; the family caregivers themselves are in great need of information and support from staff. A major point made by the researchers is, that institutional policy must view families as continued providers, as well as recipients of care and support. The researchers plan to support agency personnel in the use of the tool, and thus lead to ongoing evaluation and improvement of care.

The two latter studies dispel the myth that family caregiving is confined to the home. Demands from the family for tending and needs of the family caregivers for attention, information, support and care continue within the institutional setting.

In relation to care of children, Krulik and a group of nurses launched a major action research program on comprehensive home care following the comparative study (Krulik, Hirschfeld and Sharon, 1984) summarized above. The first step was a pilot project, co-ordinated by Krulik and Katz, geared toward identifying the barriers nurses faced in providing care to these families.

In 1984–5 a group of 28 public health nurses were selected to participate in the pilot study. Results of the pilot study led to three basic conclusions:

1. Nurses were found to be lacking adequate knowledge in regard to the content of their intervention in three specific areas:
   aspects of the disease, its manifestations and possible interventions;
   psychosocial aspects of caregivers and families;
   communication skills;
2. Lack of clarity was perceived in terms of nurses' role in regard to care of families with a chronically ill child. This was explained by the fact that their repertoire of skills and orientation had been developed around care of the healthy child and hesitation and anxiety resulted in relation to this new role;
3. Lack of professional security resulted, as evidenced by expression of feelings of inability to contribute anything special to the child's care on the one hand and on the other, 'satisfaction' at the child's being cared for by other professionals. In summary, the current level of knowledge and existing community services were found inadequate in meeting the special requirements of these children and their families.

The next step was funded by the Kellogg Foundation. The Kellogg project was developed and continues as a comprehensive home-care programme for families with a chronically ill child. It represents a conceptual move from a child orientation with the mother as the prime caregiver to a family orientation. The overall aim of the programme is the preparation of public health nurses for successful home and community-based interventions for families with a chronically ill child. The emphasis was and is on enhancing the families' independence in coping with their situation.

A training programme was developed to address itself to three aspects: knowledge, attitudes and skills. It is hoped that by the end of the programme there will be an increase in relevant knowledge concerning chronic illness and a clarification of attitudes and beliefs of the nurses and the participating families, as well as an enhancement of professional skills of the nurses and coping abilities of the families.

The evaluation component of this action research measures the above variables. To date baseline data were collected from 50 nurses and their control group, as well as from 50 families and their matched controls. The educational programme focusing on intervention models is under way.

In summary, research has shown to date, that caregiving is a common phenomenon over and above the differences of age, kind of illness, or context of care. Family care plays a major role in the patients' quality of care and life. Family caregivers are a group at risk with special needs. They can gain a lot from information and guidance related to the care they provide, as well as from on-going support for their own physical, emotional and social needs. Nurses can make a major difference in these families' lives.

## FUTURE PLANS

The above is an example of our beginning efforts to link independent studies into a meaningful body of knowledge for nursing.

The research areas these authors would like to consider in the future are:

1. The reality of family caregiving in terminal stages;
2. The ethical dilemmas related to proxy decisions in caregiving (e.g. decisions caregivers make on behalf of children or demented elderly) and the impact such decisions have upon families;
3. The links and effective mix of formal and informal support systems;
4. The effectiveness of different interventions for direct care, as well as for support of caregivers.

These and other topics are of vital interest to nursing in Israel. As in all areas, Israeli nurses invest great effort in seeking relevant questions from practice, translating them into sound research and utilizing the findings for improving nursing practice, education and the development of a sound and humane health and social policy.

## REFERENCES

Aiken, L.H. and Mullinex, C.F. (1987) The nurse shortage. Myth or reality? *N. Engl. J. Med.*, **317**, 646–51.

Bergman, R. (1987) *Research and studies on nursing in Israel.* Monograph, Department of Nursing, Tel Aviv University.

Bergman, R. and Gerstanski, Y. (1987) *Development of an Instrument to Evaluate quality of care in a psycho-geratric unit.* Monograph, Department of Nursing, Tel Aviv University.

Bowlby, J. (1982) Attachment and love: retrospect and prospect. *Am. J. Orthopsychiatry*, **52**, 664–678.

Delamothe, T. (1988) Nursing grievances, I–IV, *Br. Med. J.*, **296**, 25–28, 120–123, 182–185, 271–274, 345–347, 406–408.

Dunea, G. (1988) Nurse shortages. *Br. Med. J.*, **296**, 911–912.

Gerstanski, Y. (1986) *The impact of institutionalization of a demented patient upon the family.* Unpublished thesis, Department of Nursing, Tel Aviv University.

Hirschfeld, M.J. (1983) Home care versus institutionalization: family caregiving and senile brain disease. *Int. J. Nurs. Stud.* **20**, 23–32.

Hirschfeld, M.J., Ziv, L., Bar Tal, Y., and Sharon, R. (1984) *A tool for symptom assessment.* Unpublished research report, Department of Nursing, Tel Aviv University.

Krulik, T., Hirschfeld, M.J. and Sharon, R. (1984) *Family care for the severely handicapped children and aged in Israel.* Monograph, Department of Nursing, Tel Aviv University.

Lindenbaum, N.V. (1989) *Attachment in family care – caring for the demented spouse.* Master thesis, Department of Nursing, Tel Aviv University.

Stein, R.F.K. and Jessop, D.J. (1982) *What diagnosis does not tell: the case for a non-categorical approach to chronic physical illness.* Paper presented in the Meetings for the Society of Pediatric Research/Ambulatory Pediatric Association, Washington, DC.

# CHAPTER NINE

# Care of moderately and severely demented patients in Sweden

## *Astrid Norberg*

Health care in Sweden is a socialized system. The county councils have the main responsibility while private enterprises play a negligible role. There is a national health insurance system which covers most of the costs of the patient. A patient who stays in a hospital, for instance, has to pay 55 Swedish crowns per day out of his own pocket while the real costs often exceed 800 Swedish crowns in a psychogeriatric ward and 1100 Swedish crowns in a geriatric ward.

Sweden is one of the countries with the largest number of institutional beds per inhabitant (Grundy and Arie, 1981). In 1985 about 30% of all people 80 years old or more lived in some kind of institution (Co-ordinated Care of the Elderly, 1986). However, in the last decade big changes have been planned. There are political decisions to transfer resources from institutional care to home care. There are two main reasons for this. First, there are humanitarian reasons. The patient's integrity and dignity are supposed to be best preserved when he is cared for in his own home. Secondly, there are financial reasons. If the growing number of elderly people with health problems had needed institutional care to today's extent, tax increases would have been necessary (Lendenius, 1983).

The personnel of hospital wards consists mainly of enrolled and registered nurses. The proportion of registered nurses is growing. At the same time a modified form of primary nursing is being applied. A registered nurse and an enrolled nurse work together as a mini team. In home care the situation is more problematic. The aim is that the social services of the local authorities should help with things like cooking while home care personnel should provide nursing care. In reality, however, this is not always the case. Unskilled personnel from the social services take part in nursing care (Medical Care at Home, 1983).

In 1986 about half of the patients in home care were cared for by their relatives, often retired wives, daughters and daughters-in-law (Care on the

Quiet, 1986). An urgent question for the future is whether women will and should be willing to take the responsibility for family care. This is seen as a threat against women's emancipation (Waerness, 1983).

In 1985 17.5% of the population were older than 65 years. This figure is estimated to be 20% by the year 2025 (Official Statistics of Sweden, 1986). Compared to other countries in Europe and USA (Grundy and Arie, 1981) the prevalence of institutional care for the elderly is high in Sweden (Adolfsson, 1980). An investigation of nursing homes, homes for the aged, somatic long-stay clinics, psychiatric long-stay wards and psycho-geriatric wards in the county of Västerbotten in 1982 showed that 40% of all probands were demented (Sandman, Adolfsson, Norberg *et al.*, 1988). The prevalence of demented patients in the same type of institutions was about 60% in 1988 in Umeå health care district. The percentage of demented patients in nursing homes was 83 (Sandman, unpublished results). Alternatives to institutional care are being developed; for example collective housing and day care (Co-ordinated Care of the Elderly, 1986). Few moderately and severely demented patients are still cared for in their homes. Usually the patients are in institutions during their last two years (Adolfsson, personal communication). Thus in Sweden the care of moderately and severely demented patients is mainly institutional care.

Patients with dementia diseases gradually lose their abilities. This puts heavy demands on their relatives. They often experience that the patient's personality changes so that they hardly recognize them. 'It's my mother, but at the same time, it's not her', a daughter said (Ericsson-Persson *et al.*, 1984).

There is a considerable risk that relatives mourn the patient while he is still alive. They move towards psychological closure of their relationship with the patient (Siegel and Weinstein, 1983). They will then experience their sick relative as living dead. 'She is already dead, it is cruel when the heart goes on beating in a dead body'. This is how a relative described her experiences (Ericsson-Persson *et al.*, 1984).

Nursing research into the care of demented patients has been performed at the University of Umeå for ten years. The aim of this chapter is to describe a model of the care of demented patients developed in that research, to relate research results to this model and to discuss possible improvement of care.

According to the model (Athlin and Norberg, 1987a) the very core of caring is the interaction between the patient and his caregiver. The caregiver has to be able to use herself in a therapeutic way and deliver care systematically. The physical environment has to be adapted to the patient's abilities as has the organization of care. All caring activities should be guided by a humanistic philosophy. Education should contain all these components and present them as an integrated whole.

## PHILOSOPHY OF CARE

An important basis for the philosophy of care is the fact that the patient and his caregiver are interdependent although the caregiver has more power than the patient who is more dependent. The mere existence of the patient presents an ethical demand to the caregiver. He/she has to take her responsibility and act so that the patient's life is best promoted (Bexell, Norberg and Norberg, 1985).

The interdependence could be interpreted on the basis of the E.H. Erikson theory of 'eight stages of man' (Erikson, 1982). During life man passes through eight crises and the development depends on how he solves these crises. All eight crises are always latent in the person but during each stage of development a specific crisis becomes manifest. The outcome of one crisis affects the manifestation of the next. There is always an actual version of all the eight crises.

The demented person is still first of all a human being and should be helped to solve all his life crises as positively as possible. The experience of integrity presupposes that he also experiences trust, autonomy, initiative, industry, identity, intimacy and generativity as much as possible (Norberg and Sandman, 1988). Each single activity of care should have at least two aims: the feeding of the patient should, for instance, aim at providing him with nutrients and oral satisfaction but just as important an aim should be to promote his integrity (Norberg, Athlin and Winblad, 1987).

For each care activity the caregiver has to be creative and figure out how he/she could promote the patient's integrity. In the following only a few glimpses of what could be done will be given.

*Trust versus mistrust (hope)*. It is easier to trust a caregiver if you meet her often and she behaves in a predictable way.

*Autonomy versus shame and doubt (will)*. Although the demented patient might not be able to make decisions in complicated matters he might still be able to decide about his everyday life.

*Initiative versus guilt (purpose)*. It is more probable that the patient will take initiatives when he notices that his caregivers take them seriously.

*Industry versus inferiority (competence)*. The patient will feel much more competent when the caregiver encourages him to use abilities than when she exposes his disabilities.

*Identity versus identity confusion (fidelity)*. The caregiver has to connect to the identity that means most to the patient.

*Intimacy versus isolation (love).* The severely demented patient might be unable to interact with a group of persons but still be able to interact in dual relations.

*Generativity versus stagnation (care).* Even the demented patient can care for others when given an opportunity.

*Integrity versus despair (wisdom).* Even the demented patient has a need to experience meaning and wholeness. When he becomes stimulus-bound (Obler, 1981) the experience of meaning and wholeness has to be connected to the concrete situation. The patient could, for example, experience meaning and wholeness during a meal by recognizing the food as something connected to his past and important for his future.

Care must be organized and delivered in such a way that even the patient's relatives are given support to solve their life crises. The fact that a close relative becomes demented leads to a series of traumatic crises (Cullberg, 1975) that can lead to a revival of life crises solved previously.

An investigation of the experiences of the relatives of terminally ill demented patients revealed that the care was not organized in a way that promoted their experience of integrity (Sällström, Sandman and Norberg, 1987). The trust between relatives and personnel must be mutual. They have to feel that they can participate in decisions about care and take initiatives. They have to feel they are treated as unique persons and also feel that their relation with the caregivers is close enough. They have to feel that they contribute to care and that they get some help to connect their experience of the demented relative to their past, present and future.

The caregiver is also a human being who needs to solve her life crises at each stage of development. She cannot promote the patient's integrity if her own is not promoted. The patient's care environment is the caregiver's work environment. It should be organized so that the caregiver's integrity becomes promoted. This means that the caregiver should have an opportunity to experience trust, autonomy, initiative, industry, identity, intimacy, generativity and integrity. The notion that the patient, his relatives and caregivers have the same basic needs is a consequence of their interdependence.

Sandman (1986) has proposed a model for describing the development of dementia care in Sweden. He describes three dimensions, namely *methods*: compensation versus taking over, *means*: natural versus artificial, and *ends*: quality of life versus survival (pp. 36–39). The role of the nurse, he thinks, is to help the patient to use his abilities and structure the environment so that his actions are facilitated. She should only take over the patient's self-care activities when there are no other means to help him. Care should also, if possible, use natural means and the environment should be home-like. Drugs could for example be replaced by natural treatment such as using high-bran bread instead of laxatives (Sandman *et al.*, 1983). Compensatory and natural treatment is closely linked to a high priority given to the patient's quality of life.

The high value given to the patient's quality of life is evident in decisions concerning terminal care of severely demented patients. When the patient does not co-operate in feeding any more his caregivers themselves might feel faced with an unsolvable conflict (Norberg, Norberg and Bexell, 1980; Åkerlund and Norberg, 1985; Norberg, Asplund and Waxman, 1987). They wish to keep the patient alive by feeding him, but when they are feeding him they fear that they may hurt him. His refuse-like behaviour might leave them with a feeling that they force him. Whatever the caregiver does, she might feel that she does the wrong thing. This is very frustrating. Several caregivers, however, find a solution to the conflict by giving priority to the patient's quality of life over his survival (Åkerlund and Norberg, 1985). This contrasts sharply with the opinions expressed by caregivers in Israel (Norberg and Hirschfeld, 1987).

## INTERACTION BETWEEN THE DEMENTED PATIENT AND HIS CAREGIVER

The interaction between the demented patient and the caregiver has been described by means of the following concepts: clarity of cues, sensitivity, interpretation, responsiveness and synchrony (Athlin and Norberg, 1987a).

The patient has to send clear cues and the caregiver has to be sensitive enough to perceive them. Then she has to make a correct interpretation, be willing to answer the patient and send clear cues back that he is sensitive enough to pick up and interpret. The interaction should lead to synchrony between patient and caregiver; they seem to be waltzing.

The dementia disease involves impairments that hamper the interaction process. Memory disturbances, problems of logical reasoning, aphasia, agnosia, apraxia, paratonia and primitive reflexes make the patient's cues unclear, reduce his sensitivity and interpretation ability. The patient's responsiveness will also be impaired. He will gradually lose his ability to communicate. At each stage of the process the caregiver has to assess his abilities so that she can adapt her communicative cues to them.

The patient who can still use verbal cues might have problems to find words for things although he can demonstrate their use (Martin and Fedio, 1983). The caregiver could then try to communicate without asking him to name objects. The patient might have problems to initiate speech although he can continue once started (Obler, 1981). The caregiver could then help him by saying the first sentences. A religious patient for instance did not remember who God was when asked. But when the caregiver helped him to clasp his hands and started to pray: 'Thank you God' he continued to pray adequately (Karin Zingmark, personal communication).

In an explorative study a group of moderately demented patients had coffee together and were encouraged to talk to each other (Åkerlund and Norberg, 1986). The researcher did not initiate any topics but supported the dialogue between the patients and helped them to keep their conversation together. The astonishment was great when it turned out that the patients discussed matters like love and marriage, faithfulness, and unfaithfulness, illness and fear of death, separation. The same patients had previously been observed in a reality orientation group. In that context their verbal behaviour was more restricted. They answered questions from the group leader and looked like 'pupils who had not done their homework'. It is hard to know how to interpret these observations. A suggestion is that demented patients function better on more emotional levels than on cognitive levels. If this is the case, adapting verbal communication to the moderately demented patient might not mean to make it simple and childlike but emotionally deeper.

When the patient has lost his verbal language and gestures his face is the main source of information about his feelings. The patient, however, may send very vague and ambiguous cues. In a study of two severely demented patients it turned out that the only facial behaviour that differed significantly between periods of different kinds of stimulation was the frequency of eye blinkings and the frequency of mouth movements (Norberg, Melin and Asplund, 1986). It seems obvious that the caregiver needs considerable sensitivity in order to be able to perceive these cues. None the less a few caregivers did state that it was quite easy to communicate with the two patients (unpublished data from the study) as 'they talked with their eyes'. This of course does not necessarily mean that the caregivers reacted to the patients' eye blinkings. They might as well have reacted to changes in the size of his pupil, which was not observed in the study.

When the caregiver has perceived the patient's cues, she has to interpret them appropriately. For this reason she needs knowledge about his past history. She can sometimes deduce his wishes from his behaviour and knowledge about his previous experiences, values and habits (cf. Veatch, 1984). She also needs to be able to recognize dementia symptoms such as identifying the occurrence of primitive reflexes and discriminate them from purposeful actions. Paratonia for instance is a phenomenon that is often misinterpreted. It means increasing muscle tone during passive movements of different strength. It is often interpreted by caregivers as the patient's resisting consciously and refusing to participate in an activity (cf. Sandman, Norberg, *et al.*, 1986).

Inability to interpret the patient's cues causes serious problems in care. To assess whether the severely demented dying patient feels thirsty, is for instance very problematic (Michaelsson, Norberg and Samuelsson, 1987). The patient's inability to express clearly his need to go to the toilet is another example. In fact, the patient's difficulties in communicating seem to be the core problem that gives rise to many other problems.

## THE SYSTEMATIC DELIVERY OF NURSING CARE TO DEMENTED PATIENTS

In order to be able to provide an individualized care the caregiver has to make systematic assessments and use diagnostic reasoning (Carnevali *et al.*, 1984). This, however, is not always the case in Sweden. Interviews with nurse aids and enrolled nurses in nursing homes in northern Sweden revealed that caregivers often answered the question: What do you do when a patient does not eat?, by directly suggesting feeding actions such as leaving the patient or changing food and not by suggesting diagnostic processes (Norberg *et al.*, 1988). The caregivers for instance did not differentiate between inability to eat and purposeful refusal to eat.

When helping the demented patient with his activities of daily living it is essential to perform a systematic assessment of his abilities and disabilities. The nurse has to assess on which level of performance the patient can function so that she does not give him too much help nor too little.

Morning care can be seen as a system of self-care that could be divided into subsystems, action sequences and unit acts (Bullowa, 1975). Each of the subsystems, washing, showering, combing, tooth-brushing, shaving and dressing, consists of several parts. In an article based on observations of five moderately and severely demented patients a classification system for the assessment of the patient's self-care abilities related to morning care was suggested (Sandman, Norberg *et al.*, 1986). In order to perform complete morning care the patient has to '1. Be motivated to perform the actions; 2. Recognize and understand (his) own body: 3. Have the sensory-motor functions required for performing the actions, e.g. hearing, strength; 4. Understand the purpose of each subsystem, e.g. that his hands should be clean and dry; 5. Recognize and understand the objects used during morning care, e.g. soap towel; 6. Be able to perform the necessary actions, e.g. perform movements to wash himself; 7. Be able to combine different actions into a logical goal-directed sequence of actions, e.g. wet, rub, rinse and dry; 8. Be able to combine the separate subsystems, e.g. wash, dress and comb, into a logical whole; 9. Have an adequate perception of time and how much time to use for each subsystem; 10. Understand quality, e.g. judge if his hands are clean enough. If the patient is dependent on a nurse: 11. Be able to communicate; 12. Recognize and understand the function of the nurse.

The observations of the five patients showed that their behaviour systems were fragmented. Thus they were able to perform single acts but could not combine them into a meaningful whole. Nor were they able to judge when to stop an activity. It was, however, possible to compensate for the patients' deficiences to a certain extent. When a nurse initiated an act it sometimes happened that the patient was able to proceed automatically and finish it. In a warmer atmosphere the patient's motivation and understanding of the meaning of an activity could be improved.

## THE ENVIRONMENT

Svensson (1984) describes how changes in the environment brings about changes in the person, for example changes in ego sets, since the person constantly struggles to adapt to his surroundings. As the demented patient has a reduced ability to reorganize his ego sets he becomes extremely sensitive to press from the environment. He becomes disoriented and shows maladaptive behavior. Svensson states that is is a paradox that when the patient is institutionalized he 'is forced to give up his reality in order to adapt to a reality that is poorer but also at the same time, that has been created to cure him'.

In a study five moderately demented patients were observed during meals alone and later on together with two caregivers who were first dressed in civil dresses and then dressed in white hospital uniforms (Sandman, Norberg and Adolfsson 1988). It was obvious that the environment affected the patients' behaviour to a great extent. When they had their meals alone the two least demented patients took the role of hostesses and helped the other patients by serving them food, reminding them to eat, and correcting their mistakes. The least demented patient even fed the most demented. When the caregivers participated in the patients' meals dressed in civil dresses the least demented patient recognized them and left her role of a hostess. When the caregivers were dressed in white hospital uniforms even the next least demented patient recognized them and took the passive patient role.

## THE ORGANIZATION OF CARE

A successful interaction with the demented patient presupposes that the caregiver has continuous contact with him and his relatives. This is not always the case. In 1982 a little more than 14 000 feedings of nursing home patients were assessed in the county of Västerbotten in northern Sweden (Bäckström, Norberg and Norberg, 1987). The median number of caregivers who fed each patient during a 4-week period was 18. The number was even higher for patients with serious feeding problems. Probably the connection between the numbers of caregivers and the degree of feeding difficulty was complicated. On the one hand it seems reasonable to believe that discontinuous contacts between patients and caregivers created feeding problems. On the other hand the fact that the patient exhibits feeding problems could make caregivers avoid him.

When the organization of care was changed from a task assignment care system to a patient assignment care system during feeding the caregivers experienced that feeding problems decreased (Athlin and Norberg, 1987b). Three caregivers were interviewed after their first, seventh and fourteenth feeding of one patient each, and one caregiver was interviewed after the same numbers of her feeding of three patients. The results showed that with increased experience of a patient caregivers became more certain about how to interpret his cues, and how to adapt their behaviour to him. During the first feedings of a patient one caregiver for instance noticed that he refused to eat after a while. With increasing experience she understood that she herself elicited the refuse-like behaviour by wiping his mouth when he spilled food as it evoked search reflexes in him. When the caregiver had this insight she refrained from wiping and the refuse-like behaviour disappeared. There were several examples in the study of how some feeding problems vanished and others remained but became manageable thanks to the caregivers' improved understanding of the feeding process. Caregivers' attitudes towards patients became more positive when they understood their behaviour better.

In the care of severely demented patients it seems logical to assume that the improvement of the interaction between patient and caregiver mainly depends on the fact that the caregiver can interpret the patient's cues better and also adapt to them. Nevertheless, the above study (Athlin and Norberg, 1987b) showed that even severely demented patients adapted their behaviour to that of the caregiver. One patient for example changed from opening her mouth when the spoon touched it to opening it anticipatorily when the spoon approached it.

Even with a continuous contact between patient and caregiver it can be hard to interpret the patient's cues. In order to make sure that the patient is given care as much in accordance with his own preferences as possible it is necessary that his caregivers know about his previous life, values, opinions and habits (Veatch, 1984). Therefore they need a method to collect this information. Interviews with caregivers in a geriatric hospital in northern Sweden, however, showed that caregivers had a poor knowledge of their patients' past mainly due to their not using the methods available for obtaining this information (Ekman and Norberg, 1988).

## TRAINING CAREGIVERS FOR DEMENTIA CARE

At a hospital in central Sweden all personnel on a geriatric ward were taught how to provide integrity-promoting care in accordance with the model presented above (Kihlgren, Hallgren, Norberg *et al.*, in press). The training that lasted for five days ended by the caregivers taking a collective decision about how to change care on their ward. They then had the support from a nurse researcher and a social worker student during the intervention. The caregivers changed both the physical environment and their ways of providing care so that it fitted demented patients better. Analysis of videorecorded morning care sessions showed that the caregivers had changed their interaction with patients after the training; for instance they gave patients more opportunities to participate in activities and decisions and asked them about their opinions (Kihlgren *et al.*, 1987). The most interesting results of these changes were the facts that compared to a control group the patients improved their motoric functions and exhibited a decreased degree of confusion, anxiety and depressed mood (Bråne, Karlsson, Kihlgren and Norberg, 1989). The patients also increased their level of somatostatin in the cerebrospinal fluid (Widerlöv, Bråne, Ekman *et al.*, 1989). This finding was interpreted as an indication that the environment affects the same brain mechanisms as does the dementia disease.

There is much aberrant behaviour that demented patients exhibit and that can easily be misinterpreted. Training of personnel to interpret this behaviour can improve care dramatically.

Caring for institutionalized demented patients is very demanding work, probably mainly due to the problems of communication and the poor prognosis. A study of caregivers in the county of Våsterbotten, Sweden, showed that there was a larger proportion of caregivers who exhibited symptoms of tedium on wards with many demented patients than on other wards (Åström *et al.*, 1987). It seems reasonable to assume that a better knowledge of how to communicate with demented patients, how to organize and plan care and how to manipulate the environment will make care work more interesting. If work is guided by a philosophy of care that emphasizes that the patient, his relatives and caregivers are human beings, it seems probable that many caregivers would experience not tedium but job satisfaction.

## REFERENCES

Adolfsson, R. (1980) *Clinical Studies and Chemical Pathology in Normal Aging and Dementia of Alzheimer Type.* Medical Dissertation No. 62, Umeå University, Sweden.

Athlin, E. and Norberg, A. (1987a) Interaction between the severely demented patient and his caregiver during feeding. A theoretical model. *Scand. J. Caring Sci.*, **1**, 117.

Athlin, E. and Norberg, A. (1987b) Caregivers' attitudes to and interpretations of the behaviour of severely demented patients during feeding in a patient assignment care system. *Int. J. Nurs. Stud.*, **24**, 145.

Bäckström, Å., Norberg, A. and Norberg, B. (1987) Feeding difficulties in long-stay patients at nursing homes. Caregiver turnover and caregivers' assessments of duration and difficulty of assisted feeding and amount of food received by the patient. *Int. J. Nurs. Stud.*, **24**, 69.

Bexell, G., Norberg, A. and Norberg, B. (1985) Ethical conflicts in long-term care of aged patients. An ontological model of the care situation. *Ethics & Medicine*, **1**: (3), 44.

Bråne, G., Karlsson, I., Kihlgren, M., Norberg, A. (1989) Integrity-promoting care of demented nursing home patients: psychological and biochemical changes. *Int. J. Ger. Psychiatry*, **4**, 165–72.

Bullowa, M. (1975) When infant and adult communicate, how do they synchronize their behaviours, *Organization of Behaviour in Face-to-Face Interaction*, in (eds A. Kendon, R.M. Harris and M.R. Kay) Paris, Mouton.

Care on the quiet. The role of relatives S in the care of the elderly . (Swe.) *SPRI publication, 1986: 200.*

Carnevali, D.L., Mitchell, P.H., Woods, N.F. and Tanner, C.A. (1984) *Diagnostic Reasoning in Nursing.* Lippincott, Philadelphia.

Co-ordinated Care of the Elderly. Home, service, care. (Swe.) *General Advice from the National Swedish Board of Health and Welfare, 1986: 1.*

Cullberg, J. (1975), *Crises and Development* (Swe.) Natur och Kultur, Stockholm, pp. 132–46.

Ekman, S.-L., Norberg, A. (1988) The autonomy of demented patients. Interviews with caregivers. *J. Med. Ethics*, **14**, 184.

Ericsson-Persson, B., Galvan, S., Norberg, A. and Bexell, G. (1984) Care of senile demented patients in the final stage of the disease as experienced by their close relatives. *J. Clin. Exp. Gerontol.*, **6**, 17.

Erikson, E.H. (1982) *The Life Cycle Completed. A Review*, New York, Norton.

Grundy, E. and Arie, T. (1981) Institutionalization and the elderly: International comparisons. *Age and Ageing*, **13**, 129.

Kihlgren, K., Hallgren, A., Norberg, A., Bråne, G., Karlsson, I. (1989) Effects of training in integrity-promoting care on interaction at a long-term ward. Analysis of videorecorded social activities. *Scand. J. Caring Sci.*, in press.

Kihlgren, M., Kuremyr, D., Norberg, A., Engström, B. and Karlsson, I. (1987) Stimulating environment and kind treatment: Training of personnel and its effect on morning care of demented patients (Swe.), in *Rapport från omvårdnadskonferens i Örebro den 7–8 maj 1987.* Del 1. Örebro läns landsting – Högskolan i Örebro. Rapportserien Nr 42, pp. 104–8.

Lendenius, K. (1983) Care of the elderly in Gothenburg – a development program. (Swe.), *Socialmedicinsk Tidskrift*, **60**, 555.

Martin, A. and Fedio, P. (1983) Word production and comprehension in Alzheimer's disease: the breakdown of semantic knowledge. *Brain Lang.*, **19**, 121.

Medical Care at Home: a follow-up study. (Swe.) (1983) *SPRI publication, 1983: 155.*

Michaelsson, E., Norberg, A. and Samuelsson, S.-M. (1987) Assessment of thirst among severely demented patients in the terminal phase of life. Explorative interviews with ward sisters and enrolled nurses. *Int. J. Nurs. Stud.*, **24**, 87.

Norberg, A., Asplund, K. and Waxman, H. (1987) Withdrawing feeding and with-holding artificial nutrition from severely demented patients. Interviews with caregivers. *Western Journal of Nursing Research*, **9**, 348.

Norberg, A., Athlin, E. and Winblad, B. (1987) A model for assessment of eating problems in patients with Parkinson's disease. *J. Adv. Nurs.*, **12**, 473.

Norberg, A., Bäckström, Å., Athlin, E. and Norberg, B. (1988) Food refusal among nursing home patients as conceptualized by nurses' aides and practical nurses. An interview study. *J. Adv. Nurs.*, **13**, 478.

Norberg, A. and Hirschfeld, M. (1987) Feeding of severely demented patients in institutions. Interviews with caregivers in Israel. *J. Adv. Nurs.*, **12**, 551.

Norberg, A., Melin, E. and Asplund, K. (1986) Reactions to music, touch and object presentation in the final stage of dementia. An exploratory study. *Int. J. Nurs. Stud.*, **23**, 315.

Norberg, A., Norberg, B. and Bexell, G. (1980) Ethical problems in feeding patients with advanced dementia. *Brit. Med. J.*, **281**, 847.

Norberg, A. and Sandman, P.-O. (1988) Existential dimensions of eating in Alzheimer patients. An analysis by means of E.H. Erikson's theory of 'eight stages of man'. *Recent Advances in Nursing*, **21**, 127.

Obler, L. (1981) Review. Le langage des déments. By Luce Irigaray. Mouton, The Hague, 1973, 357 pp. *Brain Lang.*, **12**, 375.

Official Statistics of Sweden. National Centre Bureau of Statistics, February 1986.

Sandman, P.-O. (1986), *Aspects of Institutional Care of Patients with Dementia.* Umeå University Medical Dissertations, New Series No. 181.

Sandman, P.-O., Adolfsson, R., Hallmans, G. *et al.* (1983) Treatment of constipation with high-bran bread in long-term care of severely demented elderly patients. *J. Am. Geriatr. Soc.*, **31**, 289.

Sandman, P.-O., Adolfsson, R., Norberg, A. *et al.* (1988) The long-term care of the elderly. A descriptive study of 3600 institutionalized patients in the county of Västerbotten, Sweden. *Comprehensive Gerontology A*, **2**, 120.

Sandman, P.-O., Norberg, A. and Adolfsson, R. (1988), Verbal communication and behaviour during meals in five institutionalized patients with Alzheimer-type dementia. *J. Adv. Nurs.*, **13**, 571.

Sandman, P-O., Norberg, A., Adolfson, R., Axelsson, K. and Hedly, V. (1986) Morning care of patients with dementia of Alzheimer's type. A theoretical model based on direct observations. *J. Adv. Nurs.*, **11**, 369.

Siegel, K. and Weinstein, L. (1983) Anticipatory grief reconsidered. *J. Psychosoc. Oncol.*, **1**, 61.

Svensson, T. (1984) *Ageing and environment.* Linköping Studies in Education Dissertations No. 21, Linköping University, Sweden.

Sällström, C., Sandman, P.-O. and Norberg, A. (1987) Relatives' experiences of terminal care in long-term geriatrics. *Scand. J. Caring Sci.*, **1**, 133.

Veatch, R.M. (1984) An ethical framework for terminal care decisions: A new classification of patients. *J. Am. Geriatr. Soc.*, **32**, 665.

Waerness, K. (1983) Women and care. A woman's point of view on the care of people and professionalization. (Swe.) Stockholm, Prisma, in Odén, B. (1986) Yesterday's and today's family. A historical perspective. (Swe.) *Socialmedicinsk Tidskrift*, **63**, 200.

Widerlöv, E., Bråne, G., Ekman, R., Kihlgren, M., Norberg, A., Karlsson, I. (1989) Elevated CSF somatostatin concentrations in demented patients improved psychomotor functions induced by integrity promoting care. *Acta. Psychiatr. Scand.*, **79** 41–7,

Åkerlund, B.M. and Norberg, A. (1985) An ethical analysis of double bind conflicts as experienced by care workers feeding severely demented patients. *Int. J.*

*Nurs. Stud.*, **22**, 207.

Åkerlund, B.M. and Norberg, A. (1986) Group psychotherapy with demented patients. *Geriatr. Nurs.*, **7**, 83.

Åström, S., Norberg, A., Nilsson, M. and Winblad, B. (1987) Tedium among personnel working with geriatric patients. *Scand. J. Caring Sci.*, **1**, 125.

# CHAPTER TEN

# The patient in pain: USA nursing research

*Laurel Archer Copp*

## INTRODUCTION

Pain is a bond between nurse and patient. Pain management is a pact between them. All too often, the physician does not hear the pleading as he exercises his option to leave the scene. The patient and the nurse cannot leave – as much as both may like to do so. How they work out pain management agreeable to both is the *essence of nursing care.*

Pain management is clearly within the nurse's purview and something for which the nurse should be held accountable. Nurse researchers do not need to gain access to the clinical laboratory, they are part of it. It follows that it is increasingly imperative that nurses know the researchable questions and are more credentialed and academically qualified to carry out pain research. Research must then be utilized to affect practice in order to provide the patient in pain with therapeutic nursing care.

It has not always been thus. When nursing was essentially an art, medical science and nursing science undeveloped, the implication of pain on nursing practice was clear. The role of the nurse was instinctive, often appreciated, but as was the lot of the patient in those centuries, neither art nor science was effective.

As medicine became a science, and nursing sought to understand the implication of science on the practice of its profession, nursing care was a confusion of instinctive responses, often practised with guilt or seen as something that could not hurt when science failed.

Wall and Melzack (1984) indicate change is slow – 'So long as one person remains in pain and we cannot help, our knowledge of pain remains inadequate. However, there are reasons for optimism because there is at present a real increase of knowledge which comes in part from the abandonment of old concepts which were wrong and which held the subject in a strait-jacket.'

Therefore, because the role of the nurse was less understood by the person in pain and members of the health team, pain management and associated nursing care was less often effective. When merging art and science the nurse was more able, yet more discouraged from using her rapport with the pain patient as an adjunct to therapy. The result was and often is inattention to pain by members of the health team. Fortunately, nurses now use the best of science, therapeutic use of self, and appraise the ever growing body of pain research.

## MODERN NURSING

A modern and even cruel paradox now makes an impact. In what might be considered our most biotechnically and pharmacologically sophisticated age, pain management has not kept up with pain initiated by both old maladies and radically new technology. In fact with technology have come new ways of producing pain and extending life thus bringing to many persons, mornings which signify long hours of pain ahead, and the accompanying helplessness of being pushed beyond their endurance. All too often the patient is attended but his pain is not. In this chapter we will discuss domains of nursing research in pain.

It is also necessary to keep before us evidence of these complexities by extending our professional sensitivities to: (1) life pain, (2) disease-associated pain, (3) therapy-initiated pain, (4) nursing care-initiated pain, (5) research-related pain, and (6) pain associated with the patient's decision to forego treatment (Copp, 1985a).

Jacox, author of a much respected 1977 pain handbook recently (1989) stated at a national research utilization conference on pain:

'To give a brief historical perspective on pain research, twenty years ago, when I first became interested in the study of pain, there was virtually no (pain) nursing research in the literature. Wanda McDowell at Ohio State University had published a little red book that I carried around for years on how to assess patients' pain. A few years later Dorothy Crowley wrote a monograph on pain that was very useful. And then in the early 1970s Jean Johnson and I separately began to publish in the area, then Laurel Archer Copp, and Margo McCaffery. Now we have moved to the point where there is a third generation of pain researchers in the USA.'

In retrospect one appreciates the foresight of nursing research in pain in the USA of modern pioneer Crowley (1962) and associates. Their sensitivity was to patient, nurse, and system. 'To appreciate fully the potentialities in the nurse role, it is essential that the nurse be able to consider her role within the context of the system of interaction within which it operates.'

Modern nursing in modern health care settings brought a more systematic approach. The nursing process includes: assessment, nursing intervention based on scientific theory and practice, followed by proper evaluation based on established criteria. Professional nursing has demonstrated development of nursing theory, nursing science, and nursing research generated findings. The resultant effects are effective initiatives for nursing care of the person in pain.

Nurses and their health team colleagues in dentistry, medicine, pharmacology, public health, and related fields have forced attention, professional accountability and resultant changes by demonstrating their (a) interest in pain; (b) research in its causes and how it manifests itself in the body; (c) development of methods in pain management including the embracing of an integrated approach (pharmacological and non-pharmacological modalities) to pain management; (d) appreciation and improved understanding of the nature of the pain experience and the individuality of patient response to pain; (e) frankness to call for research on the effectiveness of specific pain modalities and interventions; and (f) the acknowledgment of the effect of the role of the nurse and nurse selected interventions associated with nursing practice.

## PAST DECADE PAIN RESEARCH OVERVIEWS

### International Language

Foremost we must use a common language of pain terms in order to read and write pain research and clinical innovation. Recognizing this need the International Association for the Study Of Pain, founded in 1973 and of which nurses are a part, developed a taxonomy. The most recent version (1986) with its descriptions of chronic pain syndromes and definitions of pain terms is a volume to which all nurse researchers and clinicians should have access.

### Nursing Theory and Research

Kim (1980), in 63 citations, divides research studies on pain into two disciplinary groups: (a) that of physiological theory based as well as (b) demographic and psychological variables related to pain. This article summarizes studies in which such variables as gender, personality, anxiety, depression, control, were examined.

She concluded for those studies she cited 'the pain variables suffer from lack of reliability in measures and comparability among studies.'

Called for were: (1) continuous efforts to develop more descriptive case studies of patients in pain; (2) fewer laboratory studies and more pain research in the clinical setting; (3) intercorrelations of multiple measures used in the clinical area yielding a composite index based on the degree of significance of each measure; (4) fewer bivariate analyses and more multivariate analyses producing at least trivariate hypotheses; (5) replication to maintain comparability and increase external validity and to replicate the same design in different clinical settings.

## Nurse Management and Cancer Pain

In reviewing the literature on the management of cancer patients in pain, Anderson (1982) surveyed therapeutic interventions of pharmacological and non-pharmacological types. A similar stated need for the conducting of research studies emerges. She comments on 'the lack of comparative studies to determine a cancer population that might benefit from one or more interventions, or a systematic analysis of the potential efficacy of a combination of interventions.'

## RESEARCH AND ACUTE PAIN CARE

Writing from an international perspective Peric-Knowlton (1984) reports that five major pain theories were extant in the literature. These included affect, specificity, pattern, gate control, and theory-related endogenous mechanisms of pain inhibition.

A second focus of the review is the effects of nursing interaction on patients' pain relief. The author emphasizes 'the quality of the nurse–patient relationship is of prime importance in the patient's management of pain. This relationship is basic to the effectiveness of all other pain relief measures.' Clinicians will appreciate citation of the basic work by McCaffery (1979).

Moss and Meyer (1966) interpreted that planned nursing care altered the perception of the pain-associated stimuli by changing the patient's attitude toward the stimuli. Diers *et al.* (1972) compared three nursing approaches in which the view of the patient was markedly different. Researchers concluded that when the nursing approach takes into account the whole patient it is more likely to produce pain relief. Importantly it was noted that the effect of nursing is greater than the effect of medication alone in providing pain relief.

Studies ranging from 1968 to 1981 show consistent contribution to pain relief through preoperative teaching (Healy, 1968; Voshall, 1980; and others). Singularly missing from the survey is preoperative teaching research by Dumas and Johnson (1972) which assisted in demonstrating to nurses how to bring the methods of experimentation and research into the clinical setting (Wooldridge, Leonard and Skipper, 1978). Contribution to pain research, citations in the Peric-Knowlton survey would indicate more pain studies were published in this time compared with years before. As we shall note from the next survey, not only were the pain research citations growing, the number of researchers with nursing credentials doing pain-related research were increasing concomitantly.

## Annual review of nursing research

The slow building of nursing research in pain gradually produced a collection of studies sufficient enough to merit review of 87 pain citations by Taylor (1987) in the publication listed above. This important review covered publications from the period of 1961 through 1984, giving the most complete in scope and depth survey of the contributions made by pain researchers and clinicians to date.

Organizing themes in this overview include:

1. Factors Influencing Assessment of Pain
2. Management of Pain
3. Research Directions

In this important review, Taylor asked the questions: (a) what are the major findings within the substantive areas of the research? (b) to what populations are the findings limited? (c) what major conceptual or methodological strengths and limitations exist? and (d) what do the studies contribute to nursing knowledge about pain assessment and management.

Acknowledging the strides made in nursing research related to pain, Taylor lists cautions and concerns. Replication of studies that extend the methodology by using improved controls and multiple treatment conditions are needed. There is a lack of sufficient conceptual documentation and explanation for the selection of treatment conditions. Needs in pain research include theory-building on pain conditions and trajectories, variations in patient behaviour, cognitive tools, and concepts for pain assessment.

In the next two decades, the pain research assignments to nurse researchers given by Taylor would include the conducting of studies in which findings will be cumulative, developing programmatic research endeavours, and obtaining funding for such research.

## The pain of children

One group of the at-risk populations are children. Reviews on the special pain needs of children have been done by Beyer and Byers (1985) and Eland (1985, 1988). Beyer and Byers reviewed research on pediatric pain by consequences of pain, pain assessment, the pain experience, and management of pain.

In describing a research career in children's pain and assessment tool development, Eland (1988) traces over time investigations of the differences between adult and pediatric pain; the research and clinical problems encountered in children's pain; researchable questions and tools of measurement, and aspects of children's pain yet unaddressed.

## APPROACHES TO PAIN RESEARCH

It would appear that those committed to pain management and pain research use some similar approaches to pain in spite of the fact they may be using qualitative or quantitative methods.

Nurses may approach pain research in a myriad of ways. Important to keep in mind is both depth and scope in such an investigation, as well as the fact that varied approaches often result in a wide variety of results, conclusions, and perceived implication for care of the person in pain. Careful overview would indicate a nurse clinician or nurse researcher could approach the scholarly work done in pain and its resultant publication by systematically considering the following salient and comprehensive if non-exhaustive list of approaches to pain. Not listed but to be presented later are techniques which have impact on pain research: (1) pain consensus conference, (2) pain research utilization, and (3) dissemination of findings.

## THE COPP DOMAINS OF NURSING RESEARCH IN PAIN

Domains of pain research indicate areas in which nurses have made a contribution to the literature and to the accumulation of pain research in varying degree. Unfortunately space will permit discussion of only some of the domains which are more research active. However, nurse researchers should consider all domains important and consider the dearth of research in some areas when developing blue-prints of pain research planning. An example: nurses are actively involved in natural disasters such as flood and fire and provide pain relief, yet it is little researched. Nurses are clinically active in man-made disasters bringing pain relief to those affected by every calamity from plane crashes to war, from famine to poisoning by radiation and toxic fumes. But even the resultant trauma has little associated pain research.

## Assessment techniques and tools

Since only the sufferer owns his own private, highly individualized pain experience, nurses must watch, listen, and infer, using a variety of techniques and analysing many types of data. Donovan (1989) states 'we cannot blame the lack of sophisticated assessment tools for the poor treatment of pain in our acute care institutions (Marks and Sacher, 1973,

COPP DOMAINS OF INQUIRY IN PAIN SEARCH

Pain assessment

Pain and suffering as human response

Pain and organ specificity

Pain and disease specificity

Pain and body system specificity

Pain measurement tools

Pain and time

Non-pharmocological intervention modalities

Pain and care setting

Pain in those populations at risk

Pain responses culturally expressed

Iatrogenic pain

Pain advocacy and social action

Pain and education

Multidisciplinary approaches to pain

Causes and theories of pain

Pharmacological intervention modalities

Epidemiology of pain

Pain, values and ethics

Pain prevention

Quality assessment and pain management

Pain policy

Pain politics and economics

Pain caused by environment and natural catastrophe

Pain caused by man-made error/intention

**Figure 10.1** Copp domains of inquiry in pain research.

Donovan, Dillon and McGuire, 1987). Our current research indicates that many physicians and nurses do not even ask patients "Are you in pain?" using a simple verbal scale'.

In the Taylor (1987) review, researchers using a variety of indices for concluding the patient is in pain are identified. Approaches used by pain researchers bifurcate into assessment using essentially non-verbal tools, and those who have simulated or adapted such highly verbal assessment tools as the McGill Melzack Pain Questionnaire, (Melzack, 1975). The pain assessment tools suggested for nursing assessment by Meinhart and McCaffery (1983) were the Initial Pain Assessment Tool and the Flow Sheet – Pain. These are now more widely incorporated into some nursing care settings. Nurses also often keep a simple pain analogue scale with them when assessing and reassessing patients in pain. Nurses in some burns units have developed their own assessment tools. Research is needed on assessment tools and their effectiveness in all settings. But in other settings, including even intensive and coronary care units, few if any assessment techniques are used and pain relief is considered by patient demand only.

Just as dental, medical, pharmacist, psychology professionals seek more sophisticated verbal refinements of an assessment scale, so do nurse researchers. Of some interest is the quest for the simplified, non-verbal quick assessment of pain which has resulted in the use of the visual analogue method of pain rating. Whereas verbal subtleties are sacrificed, such dedicated pain management proponents as N. Coyle, nurse, and K. Foley, physician (1987) at Memorial Sloan-Kettering Cancer Center urge the team to come together in their understanding of the patient's pain by institutionalized use of a common pain assessment tool.

Gradually nurse researchers are responding to the need for systematic conceptualization of the pain assessment process as is documented by Oberst (1978) and others.

## Pain and suffering as human response

The literature on the inferences of pain and suffering has been led by such nurse researchers as L. and J. Davitz (1981), and their several associates.

Researchers had essentially approached pain through measurement. Pain was, and often is, valued solely as a component of diagnosis. Effective nursing care requires nurse researchers to explore pain and suffering as a human response to illness, and to explicate the subjective aspects of the pain experience. As in all good research, the most valid data is elicited from the primary source – in this case the sufferer.

Patients in critical care units told Copp (1974) the nature of their pain experience and their response to it. Particularly important to this work were the follow-up explorations of external and internal locused pain coping (1985b) and development of a typology of self-concepts of persons in pain (1985c), namely that of victim, combatant, responder, reactor, and interactor.

Research on pain coping behaviours and strategies by nurses included Benoliel and Crowley (1977), McCaffery (1979), Jacox and Stewart (1973), etc. But only a few clinical research studies have investigated the efficacy of cognitive coping strategies for the attenuation of pain, usually not done by nurses. Current important exception is the work of Arathuzik (1986) who studied the cognitive and affective appraisal of suffering due to physical pain and the coping strategies and behaviours of metastatic breast cancer patients. Wilkie *et al.*, (1988) studied cancer pain control behaviours and in a current study of behavioural correlates of lung cancer pain is researching cognitive pain coping strategies.

Nurses involved in contributing to the psychology and philosophy of suffering include Battenfield (1984) who put forth a conceptual description, and Steeves and Kahn (1987) whose hospice patients caused them to explore the experience of meaning in suffering.

## Organ specificity

Research studies on pain are often organ specific: back pain, headache, kidney pain, or chest (heart) pain. Whole body systems are also used to designate pain such as cardiovascular pain, joint pain, gynecological pain, etc.

## Disease specificity

Most representative of inquiry using this domain is the study of cancer pain, with such sub-sets of investigation in benign, malignant, and terminal pain. As review of the literature would bear out, while the designation is specific the disease is not and research to cancer pain, produces a vast variety of research which is published in several types of professional journals. Nurse researchers include Barbour, McGuire and Kirchhoff (1986) who studied non-analgesic methods of pain control used by cancer patients; Zimmerman *et al.* (1987) identifying pain descriptors used by cancer and some evidence of response to Oberst's enumerating the priority in cancer nursing research (1978).

## Pain settings

Pain settings can be clinics, homes, burn units, intensive care units, operating rooms, or the delivery room, to name a few. The important contributions of Johnson (1973) could be listed under pain, children, or setting because of her work with hospitalized children fearful of pain. Johnson and her colleagues (1981) continue to make contributions especially in affecting recovery by preoperative intervention.

Perry and Heidrich (1982) surveyed burn units to determine how pain was managed during debridement, finding wide variation. They confirmed what nurses in burn units and recovery rooms urgently validate: children were given little or no narcotics, psychotropics or analgesics.

Undermedication of patients in pain was reported by the landmark study by Marks and Sacher (1973) estimating physicians ordered perhaps one-third less of analgesia for their patients than was needed.

Examining the undermedication of surgical patients and related nursing care, Cohen (1980) reported nurses were compounding the problem of undermedication for pain because they gave only a portion of that which was ordered.

The term p.r.n. has little meaning if such an order for analgesia is not carried out at all, or if patients in pain are never made aware they could have a pain medication.

## Pain measurement tools

McGuire (1984) has made an important contribution on assessment as she summarized instruments, designating the pain dimensions being measured, citing reliability and validity, and aspects of its application. In addition she has used the McGill Pain Questionnaire to assess pain in cancer inpatients.

Unfortunately nurse participation in the development, testing, and refinement of pain measurement tools is relatively unreported in the literature. An important exception is collaboration by nurse educator Mary Ellen Jeans in the McGill–Melzack tool in Montreal.

## Pain and time

All nurses have observed changes in patient's pain needs at night, yet research validating these observations is sparse. Nurses working with chronic pain patients have the access and opportunity to study chronic pain trajectories and analyse cases over time, yet little of this rich pain data is gathered or analysed. Copp (1987) identified the many roles of the nurse in chronic pain management as that of therapist, implementor of therapy, evaluator of therapy, negotiator, advocate, care planner/giver, and each one of these roles invites nursing research.

Nurses do participate in time-related pain when investigating aspects of (a) chronic or persistent pain, and (b) when involved in certain trajectories where there is remission and exacerbation of the disease and thus fluctuation in the pain management needs of the patient.

## Pain and politics

In some instances the trajectory over time is most obvious in chronic pain and/or terminal illness when pain management is critical yet when accountability is resisted not only by the health team collectively, but also as individual practising professionals. This is dramatically illustrated in the case history of a cancer patient by Strauss and Glaser (1970) entitled Anguish: Case Study of a Dying Trajectory. In the power pull between patients who need and deserve pain management, and staff who cannot or will not provide it, are the essence of power politics set against accountability.

Fagerhaugh and Strauss (1977) state: 'Genuine accountability concerning pain work could only be instituted if the major authority on given wards or clinics understood the importance of that accountability and its implications for patient care. They would then need to convert that understanding into a commitment that would bring about necessary changes in written and verbal communication systems.'

## Pain, values and ethics

Nurses are becoming more sensitive to ethical issues of which there are many in instances of inattention to pain, mismanagement or iatrogenic treatment and care which results in pain.

When pain relief is withheld, unethical decision may result by omission or commission. Meinhart and McCaffery (1983) state unequivocally, 'It is our philosophy that failure to treat pain is inhuman and constitutes professional negligence.'

## Cultural responses to pain

Culture has continued to be a centring concept for the pain inference work of Davitz and Davitz (1977). Abu-Saad (1984) studied cultural components of pain in children.

## Pain interventions

The National Institutes of Health (NIH) Consensus Conference described an integrated approach to pain management as one which combined pharmocological and non-pharmacological interventions for pain relief. The past decade has seen the use of more non-pharmacological intervention in the practice of doctors, nurses, and dentists.

Individual modalities such as touch, transcutaneous electrical nerve stimulator (TENS), biofeedback, hypnosis, autosuggestion, acupuncture, acupressure, behavioral modification, electrostimulators, surgical intervention, etc.) in individual studies are too numerous to list. However, the review of research and literature on methods of pain control by Whipple (1988) encompasses a variety of modalities.

Similarly, Donovan (1982) summarized non-invasive methods for controlling in cancer patients listing techniques and physiological effects.

### RESEARCH UTILIZATION

Until the findings are taken from the research journal and implemented into nursing practice, the patient in need of pain relief is not affected. Utilization of pain research has been a focus of conferences sponsored by the Sigma Theta Tau and for research utilization grants from the Center for Nursing Research in Washington, DC (Funk *et al.*, 1989).

### SEEKING CONSENSUS IN PAIN MANAGEMENT

Conference concerns are summarized below and will be discussed in brief:

1.  Undermedication: patients in acute pain may be undermedicated;
2.  Children's pain: children's pain is inaccurately assessed and children endure major treatment and surgical intervention with virtually no analgesia;
3.  Lack of education: health professionals do not learn proper management in their education preparation and their subsequent practice reveals they often practice by belief, tradition, and myth as much as from a sound knowledge base of pain assessment, pain management, and pharmacotherapeutics;
4.  Overmedication without relief: individuals with persistent pain may be overly medicated in spite of the fact their pain is not held within endurable limits;
5.  Undermedication: those suffering from chronic malignant and terminal pain may not receive the benefit of drugs tailored to their needs or routes of drug administration which will keep them comfortable.

## The consensus statement

The full consensus statement is printed by the US Government Printing Office and available from the National Institutes of Health (1986). Posed questions included those listed below.

## How should pain be assessed?

Emphasized was the fact that clinical assessment of the person with pain begins with diagnostic evaluation and clarification of the goals of therapy.

Variation exists between the type of pain, its cause, and the characteristics of the individual affected.

At the present time it is believed that relatively few valid and reliable acute pain measures exist. For persistent or chronic pain the use of verbal self-reporting and behaviour measures of many types were reported. These included verbal and written self-reports, visual analogues, the McGill-Melzack Pain Questionnaire, pain diaries, direct observation of pain behaviours, etc. Interpretation of data warrants sensitivity to the patient's individuality, culture, and modes of pain expression. Though assessment of pain in children presents special problems, innovation in the development of such tools was found to be vital since children in pain may frequently be undertreated. Assessment techniques that require magnitude estimates and cognition are also of limited applicability to special populations. In addition to children these populations are those who are cognitively impaired or faced with language, cultural, and educational barriers. More effective approaches to the assessment of pain in these persons deserves exploration.

## How should pharmacological agents be used?

*Acute Pain.* Data substantiating the continuing practice of under-medicating patients in acute pain has been firmly in the literature for more than a decade. Underprescribing by physicians was reported by Marks and Sacher in 1973. Documentation of the practice of nurses to give only a portion of medication ordered was researched in 1980 by Cohen (nurse researcher). Careful analysis of narcotic analgesic usage in the treatment of postoperative pain was made in 1983 by Weis *et al.* They revealed that patients received 70% of the maximal ordered analgesic dose in the first 24 hours and that physicians prescribed drugs in doses that were often inadequate and to be given at inflexible intervals. The optimal doses and duration of action of meperidine, for instance, as judged by the house staff and nurses, did not agree with the accepted pharmacological profile of the drug. Have these practices improved? Unfortunately a recurring theme for which it was not difficult to gain consensus was that too often are narcotic analgesics prescribed at too low a dose or given at too long an interval between doses. Why?

Speakers and Consensus explanations included incorrect pain assessment, insufficient knowledge of the drugs, and personal attitudes on the part of caregivers and patients alike about narcotic analgesics. Unwarranted fears of addiction appear to prevail and evidently they are attitudes more valued than patient's comfort. The danger of unrelieved pain states or damaging effects of unmanaged or mismanaged pain appears relatively absent in health care or professional education.

*Chronic malignant pain.* Research has shown that narcotic analgesics given on a scheduled basis in adequate doses is an improvement over the former p.r.n. method of physician-oriented narcotic use and nurse- or pharmacist-interpreted administration of drugs to address these pain problems.

An additional issue of concern is the development of drug tolerance, sometime improperly assessed in view of disease progression. Many aspects of practice to cope with increased tolerance were described: steroids, non-steroidal anti-inflammatory drugs added to the regimen may improve pain control without enhancing drug toxicity. Furthermore other modalities, were described.

An innovative approach to the treatment of cancer pain has been the exploration of new routes or methods of narcotic administration – continuous subcutaneous infusions, epidural and intrathecal routes, mucous membrane or transdermal absorption, oral formulation with slow release and absorption, and patient-controlled analgesia, etc.

*Chronic non-malignant pain.* People with chronic pain of non-malignant cause are a heterogeneous group with a variety of illnesses. Unfortunately relief is often unsuccessful. In an effort to alleviate the pain, drug dosage is often progressively raised to the point at which significant side-effects appear. The group called for special care to avoid overtreatment of these individuals pharmacologically.

*Individualization.* There may be marked individual variation in intensity of effect for any dose of a drug. Attention should be given to these variations in dose-response for individualizing drug choice and drug dosage for patients with pain. Among the many variations, variation in rates of drug absorption, metabolism, and excretion were cited with special recognition of differences in age and body size.

*Monitoring quality.* How accountable for pain managements are care institutions? The NIH Consensus Statement on Pain Management recommended that examination of the adequacy of pain relief for persons in the hospital or receiving services from other health care institutes and agencies should be made a part of existing quality assurance.

## How should non-pharmacological interventions be used?

Reported was more frequent use of and success with such non-pharmacological modalities as: relaxation (to address concurrent stress and anxiety); operant conditioning, modelling, desensitization, behavioral approach such as coping strategies, physical therapy, hypnosis, transcutaneous electrical nerve stimulation (chronic musculoskeletal disorders); biofeedback (headaches and painful vascular conditions); and acupuncture.

Individuals uncomfortable with or unwilling to take potent drugs for relief of pain seem more inclined to seek these non-pharmacological interventions, which may be used singly or in combination. Others may require a simultaneous or sequential combination of multimodal approaches incorporating pharmacological and non-pharmacological approaches to pain management.

## WHAT IS THE ROLE OF THE NURSE?

While the expertise of the many health team members of a variety of specialties of the medical profession is critical to the management of pain, the patient may see the nurse first, and in an around-the-clock sustained manner and therefore the nurse may be primary to identify the problem of uncontrolled pain.

The nurse can be the key link in facilitating communication between the individual and the family and other members of the health care team. In so doing, nurses, along with other health care professionals, can make a significant contribution in facilitating effective patient participation in the decision-making process.

The nurse sees various types of patients in many settings. In acute care settings the nurse occupies a central position in assessing the individual with pain, administering physician-selected therapeutic modalities, and in monitoring the condition of the person in pain. As the individual experiencing chronic pain is discharged from hospitals, nurses are in a pivotal position to assess the congruence between the person's condition, the need for care, and the community health, public health or home health resources available for the management of the individual in the non-institutional setting. If the patient in pain is at home the nurse is often the person who provides the care, maintains on-going communication with the individual and family, monitors the situation, and serves as the link with other care providers.

Whether or not the nurse practices as a member of an interdisciplinary team, the nurse may be identified as the co-ordinator of patient care. The role of *Generalist Nurse* should not be underestimated. Interventions provided include:

1. Preoperative patient education to lessen postoperative pain;
2. Nursing care plans that reflect individual medication schedules based on individual preference and activity schedules;
3. Implementation of non-pharmacological methods during actively painful events such as childbirth, burn wound debridement and diagnostic tests.

The role of the *Nurse with advanced training* should include:

1. Clinical management responsibilities such as titration of analgesics with a protocol according to the patient's level of analgesia, assessment, and participation in the use of both pharamacological and non-pharmacological modalities;
2. Provision of consultation and educational services to other members of the nursing staff, other providers, and community groups;
3. Active participation in research.

How will nurses be prepared to play their roles effectively?

It was strongly recommended that if nurses were to fulfil defined roles effectively their curriculum must include pain management. Further, it was recommended that nurses practising in nursing service, nursing education, and nursing research settings should be provided with fellowships for further study of pain management.

## What directions for future research in pain management?

Future research should be directed to:

1. Conduct epidemiological studies of the incidence and prevalence of pain;
2. Study the nature of pain in a variety of settings and with a broad range of populations as the basis of developing ethnoculturally and contextually appropriate assessment tools;
3. Develop and evaluate methods of drug delivery, including patient-controlled analgesia (PCA), sustained release formulations, epidural administration, and transdermal absorption of narcotic drugs to improve pain management with presently available narcotic drugs;
4. Continue research on endorphins, enkephalins, and narcotic receptors that show promise of producing better analgesic drugs. In addition, this research may contribute to a better understanding of the mechanisms of such nonpharmacological therapy as acupuncture and TENS;
5. Discover and develop more effective analgesic drugs with larger margins of safety;
6. Assess more fully the potential value of each of the non-pharmacological approaches to pain in acute and chronic pain states through controlled studies in specific populations;
7. Identify the specific factors associated with outcome within treatment modalities;
8. Determine the appropriateness of using existing research measures in clinical settings and to evaluate their validity as adjuncts to clinical judgement in pain assessments. Investigators should consider the special issues related to children in pain that have received less attention in the past;
9. Identify the factors that facilitate or hinder the dissemination and

implementation of up-to-date information in clinical practice in the treatment of pain.

## Consensus among nurses?

Whereas many patients receive effective pain relief, the pain of some of our patients may be unattended and unmanaged. In such instances those who assess, report, monitor, prescribe, and evaluate are not in communication with other members of the team which effects adequate or effective pain management of those in pain. The NIH Consensus Conference on Integrated Approaches to Pain Management challenged us to improve practice and accelerate our research efforts.

### HOW WILL NURSES RESPOND?

Whereas some measure of consensus on pain management was reached among members of the multidisciplinary team, can nurses reach consensus on issues in research and practice? The spectrum of pain is great as is the diversity among and between those nurses committed to its relief. These include critical care nurses, community health and home care nurses, obstetrical and neonatal nurses, oncology nurses, hospice nurses, emergency room nurses; nurses in pediatrics, gerontology, psychiatry, and all aspects of nursing service, nursing education, and nursing research who deal with pain and its management. Pain assessment, relief, and management is at the core of nursing care and has been throughout the ages. Are the lines of communication open between nurses which could facilitate consensus development, agreement on the state of the art of nursing research and practice related to pain management? From such could be drawn specific nursing research and clinical goals for the future.

### REFERENCES

Abu-Saad, H. (1984) Assessing children's responses to pain. *Pain* **19**. 163–171.
Anderson, J.L. (1982) Nursing management of the cancer patient in pain: a review of the literature. *Cancer Nurs.*, **5**, 33–41.
Arathuzik, M. (1986) *The Cognitive and Affective Appraisal of Suffering Due to Physical Pain and the Coping Strategies and Behaviors of Metastatic Breast Cancer Patients.* Unpublished Doctoral Dissertation. Catholic University of America, Washington, DC.
Barbour, L., McGuire, D. and Kirchhoff, R. (1986) Nonanalgesic methods of pain control used by cancer patient. *Oncology Nursing Forum*, **13**, 56–60.
Battenfield, B. (1984) A conceptual description and content analysis of an operational scheme. *Image: The Journal of Nursing Scholarship*, **16**., 36–41.
Benoliel, J. and Crowley, D. (1977) The patient in pain: new concepts. *Nurs. Dig.*, **5**, 41–48.

Beyer, J. and Byers, M. (1985) Knowledge of pediatric pain: the state of the art. *Children's Health Care*, **13**, 150–159.

Cohen, F. (1980) Postsurgical pain relief: and patients' status and nurses medication choices. *Pain* **9**., 265–274.

Copp, L. (1974) The spectrum of suffering. *Am. J. Nurs.*, **74**, 100–112.

Copp, L. (1985a) Pain, Ethics and the Negotiation of Values, in *Perspectives On Pain* (ed. L. Copp), Churchill Livingstone, Edinburgh, pp. 137–150.

Copp, L. (1985b) Pain Coping, in *Perspectives On Pain* (ed. L. Copp), Churchill Livingstone, Edinburgh, pp. 3–16.

Copp, L. (1985c) Pain coping model and typology. *Image: The Journal of Nursing Scholarship*, **17.**, 69–71.

Copp, L. (1987) The role of the nurse in chronic pain management, in *Chronic Pain Management* (eds G. Burrows, D. Elton and G. Stanley), Elsevier, Amsterdam, pp. 227–242.

Coyle, N. and Foley, K. (1987) Prevalence and Profile of Pain Syndromes in Cancer Patients, in *Cancer Pain Management* (eds D. McGuire and C. Yarbro), Grune and Stratton, New York, pp. 21–46.

Crowley, D. (1962) *Pain and its Alleviation.* University of California (UCLA), California, p. 6.

Davitz L, and Davitz J. (1977) Cross-cultural inferences of physical and psychological distress. Part I. *Nurs. Times* **73**, no. 15. Part II. *Nurs. Times* **73**, No. 16.

Davitz L. and Davitz J. (1981) *Inferences of Patients' Pain and Psychological Distress: Studies of Nursing Behavior,* Springer New York.

Diers, D., Schmidt, R.. McBride, M. and Davis, B. (1972) The effect of nursing interactions on patients in pain. *Nurs. Res.*, **21**, 419–428.

Donovan, M. (1982) Cancer pain: you can help! Symposium on oncologic nursing practice. *Nurs. Clin. North Am.*, **17**, 718.

Donovan M. (1989) Relieving Pain: The Current Bases for Practice, in *Key Aspects of Comfort: Management of Pain, Fatigue, and Nausea* (eds S. Funk, E. Tornquist, M. Champagne *et al.*), Chapter 3. Springer, New York.

Donovan, M., Dillon, P. and McGuire, D. (1987) Incidence and characteristics of pain in a sample of medical-surgical inpatients. *Pain*, **30**, 69–78.

Dumas, R. and Johnson B. (1972) Research in nursing practice: a review of five clinical experiments. *Int. J. Nurs. Studies*, **9**. 137–140.

Eland, J. (1985) The Role Of The Nurse in Children's Pain, in *Perspectives On Pain* (ed. L.A. Copp), Churchill Livingstone, Edinburgh, pp. 29–45.

Eland, J. (1988) Persistence in pediatric pain research: one nurse researcher's effort. *Recent Advances in Nursing*, **21**, pp. 43–62.

Fagerhaugh, S. and Strauss, A. (1977) *Politics of Pain Management: Staff-Patient Interaction.* Addison-Wesley, Menlo Park, California; p. 27.

Funk, S., Tornquist, E., Champagne, M. *et al.* (eds) (1989) *Key Aspects of Comfort: Management of Pain, Fatigue, and Nausea*, Springer, New York, pp. 3–6.

Healy, K. (1968) Does preoperative instruction make a difference? *Am. J. Nurs.*, **68**, 62–67.

International Association for the Study of Pain (1986) Classification of chronic pain and definitions of pain terms. *Pain*, Suppl. 3, S216.

Jacox, A. (1977) *Pain: a source book for nurses and other health professionals.* Little, Brown, Boston.

Jacox, A. (1989) Key Aspects of Comfort, in *Key Aspects of Comfort: Management of Pain, Fatigue, and Nausea* (eds S. Funk, E. Tornquist, M. Champagne *et al.*), Chapter 2. Springer New York In press.

Jacox, A., Stewart, M. (1973) *Psychological Contingencies Of The Pain Experience* University of Iowa Press, Iowa.

Johnson, J. (1973) Effects of structuring patient's expectations on their reactions to threatening events. *Nurs. Res.*, **21**, 499.

Johnson, J., Rice, V., Fuller, S. and Endress, M. (1981) Sensory Information, Instruction in a Coping Strategy, and Recovery from Surgery, in *Preoperative Sensory Preparation to Promote Recovery* (ed. J. Horsley), Grune and Stratton, New York, pp. 33–60.

Kim, S. (1980) Pain: theory, research and nursing practice. *Adv. Nurs. Sci.*, **2**, 43–59.

McCaffery, M. (1979) *Nursing Management of the Patient with Pain*, 2nd edn, Lippincott, New york, pp. 1–9.

McGuire, D. (1984) The measurement of clinical pain. *Nurs. Research.*, **33**, 152–156.

Marks, R. and Sacher, E. (1973) Undertreatment of medical inpatients with narcotics and analgesics. *Ann. Intern. Med.*, **78**, 173–81.

Melzack, R. (1975) The McGill Pain Questionnaire: major properties and scoring methods. *Pain*, **1.**, 2277–299.

Meinhart, N. and McCaffery M. (1983) *Pain: a Nursing Approach to Assessment and Analysis* Appleton-Century-Crofts, Norwalk, Conn;, pp. 356–366.

Moss, F. and Meyer, B. (1966) The effects of nursing interaction upon pain relief in patients. *Nurs. Res.*, **15**, 303–301.

National Institutes of Health (1986) Consensus Conference Development Statement Vol. 6. No. 3. (20 pages). For copies write to: Office of Medical Applications of Research, Bldg 1, Room 216, Bethesda, Maryland 20892 (USA).

Oberst, M. (1978) Priorities in cancer nursing research. *Cancer Nurs.*, **1**, 281–290.

Peric-Knowlton, W. (1984) The understanding and management of acute pain in adults: the nursing contribution. *Int. J. Nurs. Studies*, **21**, 131–143.

Perry, S. and Heidrich, G. (1982) Management of pain during debridement: a survey of US Burn Units. *Pain*, **13.**, 267–280.

Steeves, R. and Kahn, D. (1987) Experience of meaning in suffering. *Image: Journal of Nursing Scholarship*, **19.**, 114–115.

Strauss, A. and Glaser, B. (1970) *Anguish: Case Study of a Dying Trajectory.* Sociology Press., San Francisco, pp. 33–105.

Taylor, A. (1987) Pain, in *Annual Review of Nursing Research.* **5**, pp. 23–43. N.Y.: Springer, New York.

Voshall, B. (1980) The effects of preoperative teaching on postoperative pain. *Topics in Clin. Nurs.*, **2**, 39–41.

Wall, P. and Melzack, R. (1984) *Textbook of Pain*, Churchill Livingstone, Edinburgh, p. 1.

Weis, O., Sricvatanakul, K., Alloza, J. *et al.* (1983) Attitudes of patients, housestaff and nurses towards post-operative analgesic care. *Anesth. Analg.*, **62**, 70–74.

Whipple, B. (1988) Methods of pain control: review of research and literature. *Image: Journal of Nursing Scholarship*, **19.**, 142–146.

Wilkie, D., Lovejoy, N., Dodd, M. and Tesler, M. (1988) Cancer pain control behaviors: description and correlation with pain intensity. *Oncology Nursing Forum*, **15**, 723–31.

Wooldridge, P., Leonard, R. and Skipper, J. (1978) *Methods of Clinical Experimentation To Improve Patient Care.* C.V. Mosby, St Louis, pp. 48–49.

Zimmerman, L., Duncan, K., Pozehi, B. and Schmitz, R. (1987) Pain descriptors used by patients in pain. *Oncology Nursing Forum*, **14**, 67–71.

# CHAPTER ELEVEN

# Nursing research in Australia: development of patient dependency scales

*Margaret Bennett*

## GENEALOGY

It is fashionable for Australians to attempt to establish their family tree. The search is usually interesting and for many, origins can be traced back to Great Britain. So, too, with nursing research. In this chapter the genealogy of nursing research in Australia will be traced.

The great-great-grandmother of nursing research in Australia, and indeed in many other countries, was Florence Nightingale. Few professions can lay claim to such auspicious leadership in research at their very foundations as can nursing (McManus, 1961). Florence Nightingale was so renowned for her research that she was paid the honour (rare for a woman) of being made a member of the Royal Statistical Society (Woodham-Smith, 1950). Her research was primarily concerned with aspects of service delivery, not with clinical nursing *per se*. This is not surprising, for to her the very elements of nursing were all but unknown (Nightingale, 1860). Her energies were directed towards making the most efficient and effective use of available resources – physical, fiscal and human – in the delivery of health care. One of her most significant contributions was a classification of medical diseases (Woodham-Smith, 1950).

Her only research child – a girl – was Research in Service Delivery. The father, who else but Statistics. The child almost died in infancy and was sent to North America for her health. Late in life she made a union with the very strong line of Education. The resulting twin girls married the Science brothers, Physical and Social. The blood line went from strength to strength and in time some offspring migrated (or were transported) to Australia. Unions occurred between various branches of Nursing Research and the Sciences, Humanities, History and Education. The sub-branch of Clinical Nursing Research, strengthened by these unions, became strong in its own right. It is this branch of the family that holds the key to a strong, substantive discipline of nursing.

## DEVELOPMENT OF NURSING RESEARCH IN AUSTRALIA

### Nursing in Australia

Before examining the growth of nursing research in Australia, the place of nursing within the context of the broader health system will be considered briefly.

Of Australia's 16.25 million people, 85% live in urban regions. Around 7.8% of the Gross National Product is expended on health services, with almost half (44.6%) of the health dollar going to hospitals, mainly within urban areas. However, a range of services is available to the small proportion of the population that is situated in the vast outback, including mobile health teams, the Royal Flying Doctor Service and the use of satellite communications (Australian Institute of Health, 1988).

According to the 1986 census data, the mortality rate is relatively low (7 deaths per thousand); the three major causes of death are diseases of the circulatory system, cancers, and injuries and poisonings. Life expectancy is increasing (79 years for females and 73 years for males); fertility rates are declining (1.9 births per woman) and there is a high rate of immigration (1 in 5 resident Australians born overseas and 70% of those in Europe). The population is ageing and it is predicted that the 11% of those aged 65 years and over will increase to 16% by 2021. Health services within Australia are varied in order to meet the health needs of all citizens. There is an increasing emphasis on community health facilities, on health promotion and health education and on consumer participation in the health care sector (Australian Institute of Health, 1988).

Of the half million people employed in the health care sector, 67% are nurses. To meet the varying nursing needs of the community, there are two levels of nurse – registered nurse requiring a three-year education programme leading to either a certificate or a diploma, and enrolled nurse requiring a 12–18-month course. Basic nurse education for the registered nurse is being transferred from the hospitals to colleges and universities and the total transfer is expected to be complete by 1993. The profession of nursing has a complex structure, with as many as 30 specialties being practised.

Until recently, demand for nurses outstripped supply. Severe shortages of registered nurses restricted client access to health care facilities, especially hospitals. However, measures such as special re-entry programmes for registered nurses, recruitment from overseas and better industrial conditions, including career and remuneration structures have eased the situation. The need for nurses continues to increase, however, particularly as the emphasis on health promotion and health education increases. The profession of nursing in Australia is growing in strength and is dynamic and active in its efforts to meet the nursing need of all Australian citizens (Australian Institute of Health, 1988).

## Nursing Research

The pattern of health service delivery in Australia is, in many ways, similar to that in other developed countries, so, too, is the growth of nursing research. Initially, it was closely allied to the movement of nursing education into the higher education sector (Simmons and Henderson, 1964). In Australia this movement began in 1976, and as indicated above, is set for completion in the first half of the next decade. The growth of nursing research from that time will therefore be traced through two important sources – the national nursing journals (*Australian Nurses Journal*, AJN and *Australian Journal of Advanced Nursing*, AJAN) and the four editions of the Directory of Nursing Research in Australia – a publication of the federal Government which provides abstracts of all nursing research published and underway in this country.

## Journals

The number of research articles published in the AJN has always been relatively low. From 1976 to 1982 less than one-quarter of the original articles were research studies. In 1983 the AJAN – a journal designed for publication of substantial research studies and longer scholarly articles – was commenced. The proportion of research articles increased and is currently accounting for over one-third of all articles published in both journals.

The research can be organized into five categories. The first, consistent with the origins of research in this country, relates to aspects of service delivery – the use of resources (physical, fiscal and human), patterns of service delivery, quality assurance, etc. The second category reflects the influence of education and focuses on patterns and characteristics of entrants to, students in and graduates from nurse education programmes; evaluation of teaching methods, curriculum processes and outcomes; and comparisons between various types of programme, especially those conducted in the hospital and those in the higher education sector.

The influence of the Social and Behavioural Sciences is reflected in the third category that examines nurses themselves from various sociological, anthropological and psychological perspectives. This category also includes attention to the roles and functions of nurses, decision-making, especially clinical judgements, coping behaviours, stress development and control and the movement towards political awareness and activity and professionalism.

The fourth, and most important, area shows the influence of all other relevant disciplines directly on research into the substance of nursing, that is the nurse–client interaction. It is in this area of clinical nursing that those all but unknown elements of nursing are being made explicit. The final category is a miscellany and includes studies relating to health behaviour, historical research and the ubiquitous 'other' category.

Despite the influence of the various other disciplines on nursing research, the majority of research studies published in the Australian journals have been in the area of clinical nursing research (Table 11.1). This may reflect the thrust of both journals and is different from the pattern of studies undertaken in nursing, as reflected in the directories (Table 11.5). The latter, is more consistent with the influences shown to be associated with the genealogy of nursing research.

**Table 11.1** Number of research articles in each research category published in the Australian nursing journals 1976–1987

| Category | 1976–1982 | 1983–1987 |
|----------|-----------|-----------|
| Nursing service | 17 (23.9) | 15 (14.0) |
| Nurse education | 12 (16.9) | 22 (20.6) |
| Nurses | 13 (18.3) | 25 (23.4) |
| Clinical nursing | 25 (35.2) | 40 (37.4) |
| Other | 4 ( 5.6) | 5 ( 4.7) |
| Total | 71 (100) | 107 (100) |

## Directories of nursing research

Journal articles represent a conservative sample of published research literature. The Directories of Nursing Research in Australia provide a more comprehensive picture. There have been four editions, 1981, 1982, 1984 and 1986. An analysis of the contributors and the contributions demonstrates the trends in nursing research in this country (Table 11.2).

The second and third editions included most of the articles in the previous editions plus new ones. The format was changed in the fourth edition to include only new or incomplete studies. Although the number of articles appears to be declining, it must be noted that 104 of the studies that appeared previously were omitted from the last edition. If the format had remained constant, this would have taken the total to 276.

*Contributors.* Over the period covered by these directories, there has been a steady increase in the proportion of principal nurse researchers to

**Table 11.2** Number of contributors and contributions in directories of nursing research in Australia 1981–6

| Year | Contributors | | | Contributions | | |
|------|------|------|-------|------|------|-------|
|      | *Old* | *New* | *Total* | *Old* | *New* | *Total* |
| 1981 | — | 69 | 69 | — | 118 | 118 |
| 1982 | 66 | 45 | 111 | 114 | 88 | 202 |
| 1984 | 106 | 41 | 147 | 191 | 102 | 293 |
| 1986 | 80 | 38 | 118 | 134 | 38 | 172 |

**Table 11.3** Percentage of nurse and non-nurse principal researcher working alone and in collaboration

| *Principal researcher* | *Collaboration* | *Year* | | | |
|------------------------|-----------------|-------------------|--------------------|--------------------|--------------------|
|  |  | *1981 (n=69)* | *1982 (n=111)* | *1983 (n=147)* | *1986 (n=118)* |
| Nurse | Alone | 20.3 | 32.4 | 35.4 | 39.8 |
|  | Nurses | 14.5 | 14.5 | 14.3 | 19.5 |
|  | Non-nurses | 8.7 | 10.8 | 14.3 | 11.9 |
|  | *Combined | 10.1 | 5.4 | 4.1 | 3.3 |
|  | Subtotal | 53.6 | 63.1 | 68.1 | 74.5 |
| Non-nurse | Alone | 18.8 | 13.5 | 11.6 | 10.3 |
|  | Nurses | 14.5 | 11.7 | 7.5 | 5.9 |
|  | Non-nurses | 10.1 | 9.9 | 10.3 | 3.3 |
|  | Combined | 2.9 | 1.8 | 2.7 | 4.3 |
|  | Subtotal | 46.3 | 36.9 | 32.1 | 23.8 |
| Departments |  |  |  |  | 1.7 |

*This includes multidisciplinary teams of nurses and others.

other non-nurse principal researchers (Table 11.3). This indicates a certain maturity in the profession, as does the decrease in nurses working in collaboration with non-nurse principal researchers and the increase in collaborative work where the nurse heads the team.

As would be expected there has been a gradual increase in the highest academic qualification held by nurse researchers (Table 11.4).

The largest increases have been in nurses prepared at masters and baccalaureate levels while the number of diplomats has declined. It is disappointing to note that the majority of doctorally-prepared nurses have not continued with post-doctoral research.

**Table 11.4** Highest qualification of principal nurse researchers (%) (Directories of Nursing Research in Australia, 1981–6)

| Qualification | Year | | | |
| | 1981 | 1982 | 1984 | 1986 |
| --- | --- | --- | --- | --- |
| Doctorate | 6 (16.2) | 7 (10.0) | 8 (8.0) | 3 (3.4) |
| Masters | 6 (16.2) | 11 (15.7) | 19 (19.0) | 25 (28.4) |
| Grad. Dip. | 2 (5.4) | 4 (5.7) | 7 (7.0) | 8 (9.1) |
| Bachelors | 9 (24.3) | 24 (34.3) | 39 (39.0) | 31 (35.2) |
| Diploma | 12 (32.4) | 20 (28.6) | 20 (20.0) | 9 (10.2) |
| Not specified | 2 (5.4) | 4 (5.7) | 6 (6.0) | 12 (13.6) |
| Total | 37 (100) | 70 (100) | 99 (100) | 88 (100) |

*Studies.* Using the same five categories as above (Table 11.1), and adding a separate category of health-related studies, the effects of the genealogy can be seen clearly (Table 11.5).

Nurse education is the largest category and both this and nursing service have remained relatively constant over the years. The largest increase is in the area of clinical nursing and the changing face of nursing is reflected in this area. The remainder of this section will focus on the clinical nursing studies.

Clinical nursing research examines what the nurse does in the everyday activities involved in direct patient–client care. One of its major strengths is that it can demonstrate clearly the effects of nursing care in client outcomes. In the 1981 Directory, there were only 5 studies that related directly to client outcomes. Of these, 3 could have been classified under the quality assurance subsection of nursing service. They related to an evaluation of midwifery care as a diagnostic tool (Barclay*); outcomes of people with traumatic spinal lesions as observed through nursing care records (Kroeber); and changes in outcomes for psychiatric patients for whom nursing care plans were devised (Keane). The remaining two studies were undertaken as doctoral theses – one from a sociological and the other from an anthropological perspective. The first used grounded theory to examine the ways in which people in the terminal phases of a cancer-related illness coped with the progress of their disease, its treatment and their approaching death (Parker). Ethnography was used in the second study to understand how the involvement that aged persons had with their

---

*Many articles reported in the directories were not published. Therefore these will not be referenced. The reader is referred to the appropriate directory for details of any publications.

**Table 11.5** Percentage of studies in each major category (Directories of Nursing Research in Australia, 1981–6)

| Category | Year | | | |
|----------|------|------|------|------|
|          | *1981* | *1982* | *1984* | *1986* |
| Nurse education | 39.8 | 38.1 | 32.8 | 35.5 |
| Nursing service | 26.3 | 25.0 | 25.2 | 26.2 |
| Nurses | 18.6 | 20.3 | 21.8 | 16.2 |
| Health related | 6.8 | 5.9 | 6.1 | 3.4 |
| Clinical nursing | 4.2 | 9.4 | 10.9 | 16.2 |
| Other | 4.2 | 2.5 | 2.7 | 2.3 |

families influenced the care that they received from their families. In addition, this study developed typologies of family involvement, the world views of the aged people and the relevance of both to the delivery of care (Stacey).

In addition to these studies there were two that related to aboriginal people and were categorized under Health. The first involved a longitudinal study to prepare height and weight curves for aboriginal children in order to provide some guidance for nurses assessing growth and development in this group (Kettle). The second examined the health status of a disadvantaged group of aboriginal Australians and documented the changes in health status occurring as a result of interventions of health professionals, including nurses (Frith).

In the 1982 edition of the directory there were seven additional clinical studies. These showed the influence of the sciences on nursing research. Using a clinical trial, Lock compared Op-site dressings to more conventional methods and showed them to be not only more cost-effective, but more comfortable for the patient. A postal survey was undertaken by Morrison to determine the extent of patients' reactions to stomal surgery. A significant proportion (20% of 827 patients) indicated some form of maladjustment following such surgery. An anthropological method was chosen by Watson to investigate the careers of injured workers and determine the extent to which their information levels could control their life events.

A very small study to determine the effects of a brief education programme on the level of satisfaction for people with unilateral amputation following peripheral vascular disease was undertaken by Eadie. The results were inconclusive and no follow-up studies were undertaken. This is in contrast to the work of Morse who was able to support earlier findings relating to locus of control and anxiety levels by examining a group undergoing coronary artery surgery. A historic approach was used by

Williams to examine the changes in nursing over three decades occurring as a result of the introduction of tranquillizing drugs.

A study marginally related to clinical nursing was undertaken by James. The attitudes of three groups of parents were examined in relation to participation in a care-by-parents unit. From the recorded attitudes, diagnoses were made as to whether parents required assistance in such care. The areas in which they had resistance to such care were also identified. From a microbiological perspective, Dunk-Richards concentrated on micro-organisms growing in dextrose solutions used in parenteral feedings. She also examined the ecology of Gram-negative intestinal flora in patients with spinal injuries.

The number of clinical studies in the 1984 edition had increased by 16. A scientific approach was taken into areas such as the reliability of glucometers (Stacey) the clinical use of biochemical assays (Moorhouse), the genetic characteristics of methicillin-resistant *Staphylococcus aureus* (Dunk-Richards) and different methods of treatment for episiotomies (Barclay).

The influence of the behavioural sciences were evident in research into cerebral palsy using behavioural treatment and vestibular stimulation (Sellick) and into Down's syndrome using vestibular stimulation (Sellick). In addition, studies were made into functional illiteracy among psychiatric patients (Curry); premenstrual tension using a cognitive-behavioural treatment model (Morse); reminiscing and the elderly (Wysocki); development of an Italian language self-rating scale for depression (Croll); the effects of introducing a resident dog into a nursing home (Winkler) and the effects of sonic environment on psychiatric patients and music as a factor contribution to group therapy (Ter).

Social science methods were employed to determine substance acquisition behaviour in young males who abused over-the-counter cough medicines (Chadlek) and the experience of cancer in old age (Wysocki). An education approach was taken by Schneider to determine how well prepared primiparae were for parenthood.

There were 12 new studies in the 1986 edition. The influence of the sciences was still strong, and there was a clear trend towards examining nursing strategies in relation to client outcomes. Such studies focused on the terminally ill (Waltisbul), those suffering from constipation (Price), leg ulcers (Bennett *et al.*) and deep vein thrombosis and pulmonary embolism (Kershaw). There was an increase in the number of studies related to aspects of midwifery – effects of the delivery position on foetal and maternal outcomes (Webster and Molhysen); engorged breasts (Webster); breast feeding (Allen and Martins); knowledge levels of primiparae and thinking and learning ability during pregnancy (Schneider). In addition, there was one study that examined drug-related errors (Johnson).

Thus, during the life-time of the directories, the influence of education and the sciences can be seen on the clinical nursing studies. The focus has moved away from an application of phenomena from other disciplines to aspects of nursing to a study of nursing *per se* using a variety of different approaches and methods.

What of the studies themselves? Some are substantive, innovative and methodologically sound. Unfortunately, many would have to be described as follows:

1. Characterized by a diversity of theoretical frameworks and methods. It is rare to find two studies, even when addressing the same problem, that use the same theoretical framework;
2. Original pieces of work. There are few replications of other studies. Original studies are important, but one-off studies tend to raise more questions than they answer. There is a need for replication of nursing studies to give depth and substance in the area as well as confidence in the findings, in order to establish a sound body of nursing knowledge. The need also for such studies to be conducted on an international basis;
3. Of relatively brief duration. Rarely were studies followed-up, and there were few longitudinal studies. Many promising studies have not been developed beyond the pilot stage or 'interesting' findings subjected to follow-up and more rigorous testing of the findings;
4. Of small size. Many studies use small sample sizes thus reducing their generalizability and therefore reducing their contribution to the growing body of nursing knowledge;
5. Largely published locally. The vast majority of published research appears either in the two Australian nursing journals or as reports published in Australia.

Given these characteristics, nursing research in Australia can be described as having many of the characteristics of a toddler, that is adventurously heading off in all directions at once, wilfully independent, largely undisciplined and influenced by immediate concerns rather than long-term considerations, and not wandering too far from home.

At the time of writing, nursing research in Australia was in an exciting stage. It was beginning to emerge in its own right. Nursing Research Centres were being planned and established in the higher education sector and some hospitals and other health care agencies have appointed nurse researchers to their staffing establishments. More nurses were collaborating with each other and with researchers in other disciplines, particularly in relation to clinical nursing; nursing phenomena were being examined from both a quantitative and qualitative perspective; dialogue between nurses about clinical nursing research was becoming more common, and replication of international studies was being planned. The toddler stage will not last long. A new maturity is emerging and given the genealogy of

Australian research, this is not surprising.

The influence of the blood-lines is also evident on each of the other areas of nursing research, but will not be explicated here. The remainder of this chapter will consider the growing research literature on the issue of patient/client classification systems.

## PATIENT CLASSIFICATION/DEPENDENCY STUDIES

In the current universal climate of economic constraint within the health care sector, it is essential that nursing demonstrates clearly both the efficiency and cost-effectiveness of its services. Nursing provides the majority of services within this sector and is the most vulnerable to cost-cutting pressures. Nursing must therefore find valid, reliable and credible methods for determining the resources it requires and for measuring their utilization.

One way of doing this is to establish a patient classification system (PCS) – a system based on the measurement of how much nursing care particular groups of patients require at any time. In order to establish such a PCS some measure of patient acuity, patient dependency or patient/nurse dependency must be determined. Since the 1940s attempts have been made to classify patients according to their requirements for nursing care and to establish workload systems from these. This aspect of nursing research is still in its early developmental stages. Work in Australia has been in progress since the 1950s and has been concentrated in three major settings – hospital, nursing homes and the home care setting.

## Hospital-based patient dependency research

As in other areas of research, the influence of Florence Nightingale can be seen on PCS. Her system was simple. In the pavilion-type wards those who required most attention were placed near the nurses' station and those ready for discharge, closest to the door. This geographical classification was efficient and cost-effective. Those with high dependency needs requiring constant monitoring and most attention were placed where the nurses had the least distance to travel. This method did have some advantages, but was less than accurate in determining staffing needs. Modern architecture has replaced the 'Nightingale' wards and this geographical classification is no longer possible in some hospitals.

The two most common classification systems in use are termed proto-type and factor evaluation. The prototype system allows for definition of standard profiles or stereotypes of broad categories, to which a 'best-fit' criterion is applied to each individual patient/client. The most widely known example of this type is the categorization ranging from minimal through to intensive care, more often with three to five categories. In contrast the factor evaluation system focuses on individual factors or criteria which are considered critical to patient care. Each factor is defined precisely, scored, and then the sum of the scores determines the level of dependence and hence the category of care.

Each system represents an important attempt at classification. There are a number of limitations that have been identified. The prototype system was established before technology had been developed to the stage where it enabled patients to live to the extremes of high dependency, and thus under-represents this level of care (Gliddon, 1987). It allows for considerable interpretation and subjectivity on the part of the nurse, and hence both inter- and intra-rater subjectivity can be marked. There is also a tendency to overclassify patients/clients (Jenkins, 1983). Further, the decision-making process tends not to be documented. In contrast, the factor evaluation system requires complex documentation and is extremely time-consuming (Gliddon, 1987). Questions can be raised about the method of selecting and weighting the factors and Jenkins suggests that the range of indicators may be too narrow. The emphasis on objectivity may have resulted in insufficient account being taken of more subjective factors such as psychosocial support and teaching, and Gliddon indicates that more complex and technical procedures are under-represented. Both systems appear to have difficulty in providing mechanisms for determining the level of skill required of the nurse and they tend to support what is, rather than what ought to be (Jenkins, 1983).

Australian pioneer studies in this area have been summarized by Cuthbert (1983). Various methods have been used including time studies (Chislett, 1973); work sampling (Repatriation Hospital, 1962; Cabban *et al.*, 1974; Hodgkinson, 1979); activity study (NSW Division of Health Services Research, 1971) and activity sampling (Health Commission of Victoria, 1979). Two of these studies used a geographic approach, three were prototype studies with three to five categories and the remainder were factor evaluation systems with three classes (Cuthbert, 1983).

A number of overseas PCSs have been tested for Australian conditions. The most popular system has been the Rush Medicus Patient Classification System (Jelinek *et al.*, 1974; Haussman, Hegyvary and Newman, 1976). Currently, it is being used in both an unmodified and modified form in various hospitals in Victoria (McClelland, 1985). It was tested and adapted to Australian conditions in Western Australia (Martin and Stewart, 1982) and then used to compare primary and non-primary care nursing units (Martin and Stewart, 1983). It has been further tested, modified and implemented in five hospitals in NSW (Cuthbert, 1983, 1984) and tested, modified and implemented in a large hospital in the Australian Capital Territory (Scott, 1982).

There is no doubt that the Rush Medicus Patient Classification System is one of the best known PCS to come out of the USA. It is based on a number of critical indicators of care, organized into three sections – conditions, basic care and therapeutic needs. These are scored for each patient on a per shift basis and the scores indicate the type of care required – minimal through to intensive care. A workload index can then be formulated, using not only direct time, but also indirect care activities which are added as a constant factor. Quality assurance measures are also built in for each dependency level. The claim that is a reliable system has been supported by Australian data. One distinct advantage of the system is its ability to allow ratios and times to change without altering basic validity and reliability.

The PETO (Poland, English, Thornton and Owens, 1970) system has been tested in Tasmania in a major teaching hospital. This system measures nursing care requirements in clinical care units. A clinical care unit is estimated as being equivalent to 9.4 minutes of nursing time (7.5 minutes direct and 1.9 minutes indirect care). Classification was based on 10 categories, each with a number of criteria. A refinement to this system has attempted to weight staff according to their level of experience, thus giving a skills component, or quality of staffing index.

Another system which has had extensive testing here is the American Community Systems Foundation (CSF). A number of studies in NSW (e.g. Cabban, 1980) and Victoria (Williams, 1977) showed one of the attractive elements of this system for management, namely its ability to show overstaffing.

The Patient Assessment Information System (PAIS) has been developed and is being widely applied in Australia (Hovenga, 1985, 1986). It is a patient dependency and a nursing management information system. It was derived largely from the use of work sampling techniques, but included convenience data collection relating to patient characteristics, nursing interventions and occasionally quality of care. It includes criteria not only for nursing care requests (predicted) but also takes into account the presence of patient characteristics that increase the difficulty and therefore the time required for such care. It uses a point scoring method, working on the premise that the more nursing intervention required, the more dependent the patient. A productivity index can be determined to monitor the staffing situations that are either under or over the predicted level. The system has been designed for general care areas but has limited use in the high dependency units.

Although the system was designed and tested in Victoria, currently extensive testing, modification and application is being undertaken in several hospitals in NSW (Cuthbert, personal communication). The aim is to endeavour to use a system that has been developed for Australian conditions and that is widely applied.

## Nursing home dependency studies

On the basis that the care required in a nursing home setting was different from that of a hospital, two different systems have been developed in Australia for this setting.

*Benecs.* This system was developed over five years initially at the then Bendigo Home for the Aged in Victoria (1979–1981), and further tested in conjunction with the Extended Care Society of Victoria (1983–1984). During this time it was tested successfully in 22 extended care facilities in both Victoria and South Australia.

It is a scored system for direct patient/client care and on the basis of the score a category is allocated and staffing based on the average time for care for that category is calculated. Unlike the hospital systems, this one has considerable emphasis on indirect and collective care activities. Indirect care is apportioned on the basis of a very simple table relating to the size and type of ward (e.g. short or long stay) and the presence, or otherwise of nursing students. Extensive timing studies and testing of the resultant categories was undertaken to ensure its reliability and validity. It is of interest to note that staffing needs are estimated three monthly, rather than daily and that the documented nursing care plans used for the purpose must be accurate.

Although beyond the scope of this chapter, there are some interesting differences between the Benecs system and that developed by Rhys Hearn (described below). Benecs' times and frequencies of critical indicators were derived from work observations, whereas Rhys Hearn incorporated into her criteria, a base-line care policy or standard which could be changed according to the facility in which the package was being used. Rhys Hearn also allows for interactions of patient characteristics whereas the Benecs assumes them.

*Rhys Hearn Nursing Workload Package.* The original work for this package was undertaken in Great Britain (e.g. Rhys Hearn, 1972) but two major studies have been done in Australian nursing homes in three Australian states (Rhys Hearn and Rhys Hearn, 1985; Rhys Hearn, 1986).

The package enables the calculation of nursing workload for a group of elderly, disabled people in a nursing home at an agreed standard of care. The base-line care policy allows for the user to select four parameters, the actual items of care to be delivered and their frequency of delivery, the skill-level required to perform the items (registered nurse, enrolled nurse) and the method of care delivery. This means that any standards can be set, from minimum to optimum. Indirect care measures have been built into these packages, but in the latest (1986) only direct care measures are used, although collective activities are carefully described. The description of the critical indicators of care has been developed in several studies, in different countries. Those in Great Britain and Australia are similar, although the greatest area of difference relates to the indirect care measures. Computer programs are available for both the Benecs and the Rhys Hearn package.

Both these PCSs represent innovative and important work for an area that for too long has been staffed on a less than scientific basis. With the predicted growth in the aged population, such measures are essential if we are to continue to provide quality care to the senior citizens in every country.

*Visiting nurse service dependency study.* Given some similarities between the elderly in a nursing home and those at home, the Rhys Hearn package was applied to a visiting nurse facility in Western Australia (Rhys Hearn and Gliddon, 1983) and it was adapted in a two-state study by Gliddon in 1987. In this study, Gliddon compared five different well-known functional assessment tools, namely the Katz Index of ADL (Katz *et al.*, 1963); the Barthel Index (Mahoney and Barthel, 1965); the Kenny Self-care Evaluation (Schoening *et al.*, 1965; Schoening and Iverson, 1968); the Rapid Disability Rating Scale (Linn, 1967) and the OARS Multidimensional Functional Assessment Questionnaire, developed at Duke University between 1972 and 1978. The aim was to establish the 'critical indicators' of care for the elderly patients/clients. The outcome of the study led the author to develop a single tool for data collection within the Rhys Hearn package. A further comparison was made with the Benecs and Rhys Hearn systems and there was high correlation between factors relating to low and moderate dependency, but some significant differences between the two systems for those of high dependency. Extensive timing studies were undertaken of items of care and attention paid to items that were specific for home care as opposed to nursing home care. The resultant Domicilary Patient Dependency Nurse Workload Package was shown to be both valid and reliable. Five dependency groups were clearly established, from low to high, with the highest group requiring 120 minutes of direct care per day. It was also shown to be a useful information management system.

This innovative and extremely detailed study has shown clearly the levels of dependency of persons being cared for at home, and the nursing care required. It has had another value. It has shown clearly that beyond a certain level of dependency it is not possible to care for people at home and maintain a satisfactory quality of life for both the person in care and the carers.

## CONCLUSION

Research into Patient Care Systems in Australia, as in other countries, is still in its infancy. Growth has been demonstrated by the meticulous testing and adaptation of already established systems and the development of new ones specific to areas of nursing and to Australian conditions. There are many unresolved issues in this area, not the least of which is the relationship of PCS to diagnosis-related groups and other methods of payment. Currently Cuthbert is testing the notion that payment should be tied to standards, but this work is still in the very early stages (Cuthbert, personal communication).

Whatever the future, one thing is certain. In all countries nurses have to provide some means of demonstrating to other professions that they are both efficient and cost-effective in relation not only to quality of care, but in their use of those ever dwindling resources.

Nursing research in Australia is at an exciting stage. Australia has an interesting genealogy. The influence of other disciplines can be seen in each of the areas of research identified here. The focus in this chapter has been on clinical research and the nursing service area of PCS. Both these areas suggest that the toddler stage is fast being surpassed. More substantive studies into the very elements of nursing, using not only methods from other disciplines, but using those that are beginning to emerge within the discipline of nursing itself are being developed. The innovation and creativity of Australian researchers has always been evident. It will grow in the next decade as nursing research matures into early adulthood.

## REFERENCES

Australian Institute of Health (1988) *Australia's Health*, Australian Government Publicating Service, Canberra.

Bendigo Home and Hospital for the Aged inc. (1981) *Patient Nurse Dependency.* Report of Study undertaken 1981. Bendigo Home and Hospital for the Aged.

Cabban, P.T. (1980) *Patient Dependency Classification.* Community Systems Foundation (Australasia), Sydney.

Cabban, P.T., Brown, A.A., Hope, J.M. and Williams, M.J. (1974) *Hornsby and District Hospital Nurse Utilization Study Report.* Community Systems Foundation (Australasia), Sydney.

Chislett, E. (1973) *Staffing of Public Hospitals.* Unpublished working paper, Department of Health, NSW.

Commonwealth Department of Health (First, Second, Third and Fourth Editions 1982, 1983, 1984, 1986) *Directory of Nursing Research in Australia.* Commonwealth of Australia, Canberra.

Cuthbert, M. (1983) *Patient Classification for Nurse Staffing.* Australian Studies in Health Service Administration. No. 52.

Cuthbert, M. (1984) Problems in the Design and Quantification of Public Opinion Survey for the Purpose of Evaluating Patient Care, *Aust. Nurses J.*, **13** no. 8, 36–38.

Duke University Centre for the Study of Aging and Human Development (1978)

*Multidimensional Functional Assessment: The OARS Methodology,* 2nd edn, Durham, NC.

Extended Care Society of Victoria and Bendigo Home and Hospital for the Aged (1983) Hardy, V.M., Capuano E. and Spiers, B. *Patient Care Analysis,* (1985) Hardy, V.M., Capuano E., Lennon, G., Lorimer, J. and Spiers, B. *Patient Care Analysis.*

Gliddon, T. (1987) *Patient Dependency in Domiciliary Nursing.* Royal District Nursing Service, Melbourne.

Haussmann, R.K.D., Hegyvary, S. and Newman J.F. (1976) *Monitoring Quality of Nursing Care: Part 2. Assessment and Study of Correlates.* Bethesda, US Department of Health, Education and Welfare, DHEW Publications no. (HRA) 76-7.

Health Commission of Victoria (1979) *A Pilot Project of Nurse/Patient Dependency.* Division of Management Services, Melbourne.

Hodgkinson, A.S. (1979) *Progress Report of Patient-nursing Hours Dependency Study.* Health Management Consultants, Sydney.

Hovenga, E. (1985) *Patient Assessment Information System (PAIS).* Health Department of Victoria.

Hovenga, E. (1986) *Patient/Nurse Dependency Classification – Why Use It and What Is It?* Discussion Paper, Health Department of Victoria.

Jelinek, R.C., Haussmann, R.K.D., Hegyvary, S. and Newman, J.F. (1974) *A Methodology for Monitoring Quality of Nursing Care.* US Department of Health, Education and Welfare, DHEW Publication no. (HRA) 76.

Jenkins, E. (1983) Nurse Staffing Methodologies: The Relationship between Quality and Cost *Aust. J. Adv. Nurs.,* **1** no. 1 6–12.

Katz, S., Ford, A.B., Moskowitz, R.W. *et al.* (1963) Studies of illness in the aged, the Index of ADL: Standardised measure of biological and psychosocial function. *JAMA,* 185.

Linn, M.W. (1967) A rapid disability rating scale. *J. Am. Geriatr. Soc.,* **15**, 211–214.

McClelland, J.E. (1985) *Report of Commission of Inquiry into Nursing in Victoria,* Victorian Government Printer.

McManus, R.L. (1961) Nursing Research – Its Evaluation. *Am. J. Nurs.* **57** (11), 276–282.

Mahoney, F.I., and Barthel, D.W. (1965) Functional evaluation: The Barthel Index. *Rehabilitation,* **14**, 61–65.

Martin, P.J. and Stewart, A.J. (1982) Assessment of nursing care quality. *Aust. Nurses J.* **12**, no. 1, 44–46.

Martin, P.J. and Stewart, A.J. (1983) Primary and non-primary nursing – evaluation by process criteria. *Aust. J. Adv. Nurs.,* **1** no. 1, 31–37.

NSW Division of Health Services Research (1971) *Report of Nursing Activities, Hornsby and District Hospital.* Health Commission of New South Wales, Sydney.

Nightingale, F. (1860) *Notes on Nursing: What it is and What it is not.* Dover Inc., New York.

Poland, M., English, N., Thornton, N. and Owens, D. (1970) PETO A System for Assessing and Meeting Patient Care Needs. *Am. J. Nurs.* **70** (7) 1479–1882.

Repatriation Hospital (1962) *Study of Ward Nursing Activities in Repatriation*

General Hospitals: Concorde NSW, Heidelberg Victoria, Greenslopes, Queensland. Melbourne: Repatriation Hospital.

Rhys Hearn, C. (1972) Evaluating patients nursing needs. *Nurs. Times*, Occasional Paper, April 27 pp. 65–68.

Rhys Hearn, C. and Gliddon, T. (1983) Adaptation of Rhys Hearn Nursing Workload Package to Calculate District Nurses Workload in *Health/Social Services for the Elderly and the Disabled* (ed. C. Tilquin) (Proceedings SYSTED 83, First Int. Conf. on Systems Science).

Rhys Hearn, C., and Rhys Hearn, C.J. (1985) *A Study of Patient Dependency and Staffing in Nursing Homes for the Elderly in Three Australian States.* Unit of Clinical Epidemiology, University Department of Medicine, QEII Medical Centre, West Australia.

Rhys Hearn, C. (1986) *Quality Staffing and Dependency: Non-Government Nursing Homes*, Department of Community Services, Australian Government Publishing Services, Canberra.

Schoening, H.A., Anderegg, L., Bergstrom, D. *et al.* (1965) Numerical Scoring of Self-care Status of Patients, *Arch. Phys. Med. Rehabil.*, **46**, 689–697.

Schoening, H.A. and Iverson I.A. (1968) Numerical Scoring of Self-Care Status: A Study of the Kenny Self-Care Evaluation, *Arch. Phys. Med. Rehabil.*, **49**, 221–229.

Scott, W.D. (1982) Recommended Methodologies for Determining Nurse Staffing Levels. Capital Territory Health Commission, Establishment and Review Section.

Simmons, L.W. and Henderson, V. (1964) *Nursing Research: a Survey and Assessment.* Appleton-Century-Crofts, New York.

Williams, M.A. (1977) Quantification of Direct Nursing Care Activities *J. Nurs. Admin.*, **7** (10), 15–18, 49.

Woodham-Smith, C. (1950) *Florence Nightingale*, Constable, London.

# CHAPTER TWELVE

# Transition to a qualified nursing workforce in New Zealand: a challenge for workforce planning

*Marion R. Clark, Philippa J. Moore and Elaine Y.N. Wang*

## INTRODUCTION

In the last 15 years, nursing education and nursing practice in New Zealand have undergone a major transformation. Nursing education has moved from hospital-based, service-oriented programmes to the general system of education. At the same time, the nursing workforce has changed from being one of largely unqualified (students and hospital aides) to one which is now mainly qualified. That is, it is made up of first level, registered nurses (with three years' training) and second level, enrolled nurses (with one year training). This development has had major implications for nursing practice (particularly in hospital settings), and for the structures, systems and general work environments which have such a major effect on recruitment and retention.

By the early 1960s it was apparent that there were significant problems in the system of nurse training. There was general concern that the hospital-based training programme was not adequate to produce nurses with a broad knowledge base, focused on health as well as illness, who would function effectively in a variety of different settings and would best meet the needs of a rapidly changing health care system.

After considerable activity during the 1960s and early 1970s, including three major reviews and reports, pilot schemes were finally established in technical institutes in 1973. This began the transfer of nurse education from hospitals to tertiary educational institutions (technical institutes), leading to comprehensive nurse registration.

Prior to the transfer of nursing education there were six different types of basic nursing programmes. These were general and obstetric, psychiatric, psychopaedic (mental handicap), male, community nursing and obstetric nursing programmes, the latter three programmes having been phased out over time. The new comprehensive courses combined the general/ obstetric, psychiatric and psychopaedic components into one course.

Today, in 1989, the transition is largely complete, with the few remaining hospital schools having taken in their last intakes. There are fifteen technical institutes offering these comprehensive nursing courses.

Over the period 1975 to 1987 the qualified nursing workforce has risen from 41% to 80% in general hospitals, and from 39% to 51% in psychiatric and psychopaedic hospitals (Department of Health, 1987a). This transition to a predominantly qualified nursing workforce has brought with it new priorities and challenges for workforce planning.

Against the above background, this chapter will explore the link between policy development related to these changes in education and practice over the fifteen-year period, and the research, reviews and data collection that were required to support it. It is really a case study in workforce (manpower) planning. Little organized workforce planning had existed prior to this period, it was essential for the smooth transfer of nursing education and the transition to a qualified workforce. It is now a well-refined and fundamental part of planning and policy development. The focus of early workforce studies related to problems of nursing education and determined the numbers needed in a new system that was not service-based. Gradually, however, the primary focus changed from education to nursing service as the transition to a qualified workforce gained momentum.

We have identified five clear phases of workforce studies over this period of change, and the previous decade:

1. Attrition studies relating to nursing education. This was mainly in the 1960s when work was done on attrition (and its causes) from hospital-based training programmes.
2. The development of a data base for the nursing workforce. This began in the late 1970s, when it became apparent we did not have an adequate data base to determine retention and enable us to make projections about requirements and supply of nurses.
3. The development of a model for nurse workforce planning from the early 1980s. This enabled supply projections to be made and requirements to be reassessed.
4. Recruitment and retention studies relating to nursing service. These studies in the mid 1980s focused on areas such as recruitment, retention and worklife patterns.
5. Qualitative aspects of nursing workforce planning. We are just beginning this phase, which will lead us into areas concerned with the scope and function of nursing and the appropriate level and mix of staff in different settings.

Throughout each of these phases, a constant thread has been the need to continually adapt and develop the data base for the nursing workforce. The second phase, as outlined above, must therefore be viewed as being integrated throughout the other phases.

These different workforce studies will now be described in more detail. The planning and policy needs that gave rise to them and to developments in workforce planning will be discussed. We will attempt to link the process of workforce planning to policy formulation, but the main purpose will be to describe the role of research and research-related activities in the developments that have taken place.

## NEW ZEALAND AND ITS HEALTH CARE SYSTEM

New Zealand is a small South Pacific country of temperate climate and consists of two major islands. Its area of 267 254 square kilometres (similar to that of Great Britain or Japan) supports a population of 3.3 million (Department of Statistics, 1988a). Most of the population are of British descent. The Maori people, of Polynesian origin, are the 'tangata whenua' (people of the land) or original settlers and comprise 8.8% of the population (Department of Statistics, 1988b).

'The health services are the responsibility of a partnership of central and local government; private organizations and individuals; voluntary groups and private citizens with the Government providing encouragement, financial assistance and incentives and assuming final responsibility.' (Department of Statistics, 1988c).

The State is the major funder and provider of health care. Through its district health development units, the Department of Health has been the main provider of health protection, health education and health promotion services. Curative services (inpatient, outpatient and domiciliary services) have been largely provided by locally elected hospital boards, funded by the government.

The nation's health services are currently being reorganized to integrate preventive and curative services and to rationalize service delivery on a regional basis. This reorganization is taking place in progressive stages. Area health boards, predominantly elected, are being established to administer the regional integrated health service.

As at March 1987, there were the equivalent of 29 517 nurses working full-time (38 566 actual nurses) in New Zealand. The majority of qualified nurses (85%) were employed in the three main types of hospitals: general and obstetric (65%), psychiatric and psychopaedic (10%), and private (10%). Fifteen per cent of the total qualified staff worked in community health settings (Department of Health, 1987a).

Figure 12.1 describes the pattern of deployment of qualified nursing staff across different employment sectors.

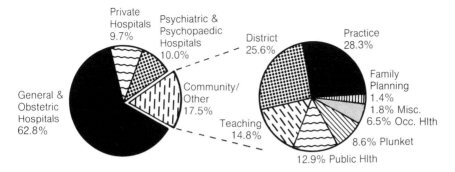

**Figure 12.1** Deployment of qualified nursing staff.

## A STRUCTURE FOR NURSE WORKFORCE PLANNING: DEPARTMENT OF HEALTH INITIATIVES

Early studies relating to nursing training, student attrition and the examination system, were carried out within the Division of Nursing in the Department of Health using, in part, data available through the registration board for nurses. The responsibility for planning and overseeing the transfer of nursing education also came under the Nursing Division. The Nurses and Midwives Board (previously a part of the Department of Health) was disbanded in 1971, and legislation (New Zealand Statute, 1971) established a separate registration authority, the Nursing Council. Consequently, new mechanisms for securing workforce data were required.

Early nursing workforce planning research around the mid 1970s was initiated by the Nursing Research Section within the Management Services and Research Unit of the Department of Health. This research and data collection continued in that structure until 1982, when the Division of Nursing was expanded to include nursing workforce planning. Overall, the Division of Nursing within the Department maintained an oversight of central policies and national issues related to nursing services and the workforce.

Reorganization of the Department of Health in 1986 resulted in a new structure which allowed for a clear focus on workforce development activities for the variety of occupational groups. A new Workforce Development Group was created, its role encompassing the three functions of workforce planning, production and management. Its broad mission is to take a leading role in the development of the New Zealand health workforce and to ensure the availability of suitable health professionals to meet the overall needs of the health services. The reorganization brought together the two aspects of research and policy and facilitated a continuing dialogue between policy-makers, planners and researchers.

The Workforce Development Group administers a special fund set up by the Minister of Health in 1985. The Workforce Development Fund provides funding for research into key issues in the health workforce, training programmes directed at particular workforce issues and priorities, and developing workforce skills in priority areas. Since the inception of the Fund, a number of studies into key nursing workforce issues have received funding support. These will be dealt with in later discussion.

## Attrition studies relating to nursing education

Major problems with the hospital-based system of nurse training began to surface in the mid 1960s and centred on increasing student attrition. At that time hospital services were expanding rapidly and student nurse numbers were increased in order to meet the demands of growing services. The service requirement of hospitals often had priority over other considerations in the selection of students.

Analysis of Health Department data for the 1960–64 period showed that only 61% of students who passed their first-year examination ultimately graduated. Of those leaving before completing training, over half either could not manage the theoretical content (28% of all leaving) or left for marriage (24%) (Department of Health, 1986). The other main reason given by leavers was dislike of nursing. The wastage rate amongst student nurses became a national concern. This high student attrition rate continued into the late 1960s. Forty-five per cent of students failed to complete the three-year programmes in 1969 (Department of Health, 1986c).

In 1965 the state final examination saw an unprecedented failure rate which finally called for a major review of the examination system. Contrary to the common belief that the examination system was flawed, evidence suggested that the problem actually arose from the period of training, particularly the inadequate education background of students and associated learning difficulties (Department of Health, 1986d).

The results of this early data analysis highlighted the need for changes to the system of nursing training. This in turn was reinforced by changing trends in health care delivery. It was acknowledged that many training schools in the past had been set up to meet service needs. There were, by 1969, 62 nursing schools offering 139 programmes. Of the 35 schools offering the three-year general programme, 17 were attached to small hospitals with less than 200 daily average occupied beds (Department of Health, 1986e). This posed further problems in terms of the range of clinical experience available for students, and difficulty in the recruitment of suitable students and qualified teaching staff.

An analysis of the levels of student withdrawals and examination failures demonstrated that the existing system for preparation of nurses was unsatisfactory and an uneconomic use of resources. Changes were urgently needed.

These findings on student attrition finally prompted a comprehensive review of nursing education. The Carpenter report published by the Department of Health in 1971 arose out of a World Health Organization short-term consultancy (Carpenter, 1971). It recommended that hospital-based three-year programmes be phased out and nursing education be developed within the general system of education. This was subsequently adopted as policy and pilot schemes for the first technical institute-based three-year comprehensive courses were established in 1973. A gradual transition over 10 to 12 years was advised in order to minimize possible adverse effects on the nursing workforce (Department of Education, 1972).

Since 1973, attrition rates of students have undergone major improvement. Eighty-seven per cent of the 1982 intake of comprehensive students in technical institutes entered year 3 of the course (Department of Health, 1987b). This compared with an overall average of 76% for intakes into the hospital-based programmes in the same year (Department of Health, 1986g). Hospital-based psychiatric and psychopaedic programmes typically had a higher student attrition rate than general and obstetric programmes.

Results from early studies on student wastage can therefore be seen as an impetus in effecting changes in nursing education and related policy development. Subsequent improvement in the attrition rate of comprehensive students after the transfer has helped to reaffirm the place of nursing education within the general system of education.

## Development of a data base for the nursing workforce

The need for a centralized data base for the whole nursing workforce in New Zealand arose out of the transfer of nursing education from hospital-based training programmes to technical institute courses.

Prior to this transfer hospital boards monitored their own student intake levels to ensure adequate staffing. With the transfer to technical institutes, annual student intake numbers needed to be determined nationally. This was necessary for several reasons. As more qualified nurses were required to replace nursing students over a period of time, careful planning of the timing and phases of the transfer were necessary to avoid disruptions to nursing services. As the government began to take over direct responsibility for the funding of these training schools, approval was required for each phase of the transfer in terms of student intake numbers and the necessary funding.

The phasing out of hospital-based programmes also highlighted the need for more information about the numbers and levels of qualified nurses required as a 'replacement factor' for the declining student numbers in hospitals, to provide efficient nursing services.

During the initial stages of the transfer, the Department of Health estimated that an annual output of 1000 comprehensive graduates would be necessary to fulfil requirements for registered nurses once the transfer was complete. In the absence of adequate data and planning methods, this was an 'educated guess' based on trends in nursing education and employment.

In 1977 a workshop on nursing workforce planning was held with the objectives of developing an integrated nursing workforce plan and reviewing the existing production and deployment of nurses in New Zealand. In preparation for the workshop, a survey was carried out by the Department of Health's Nursing Research Section, seeking information from hospital boards about the numbers and categories of nurses employed in institutions under their jurisdiction (Department of Health, 1979).

Despite the information yielded by the survey of hospital boards and other *ad hoc* studies, it was evident to the 1977 workshop that the grave lack of workforce data precluded the formulation of a national nursing workforce plan. A major outcome of the workshop therefore was a recommendation that top priority be given to developing a valid and reliable information base for the nursing workforce (New Zealand Nursing Education and Research Foundation, 1977).

Following the workshop, major effort was initiated to collect relevant workforce data. This resulted in the first census carried out in 1980 by the Nursing Research Section of the Department of Health which was to become an annual exercise. Information on staffing levels, patterns of deployment and mix of staff was sought from most employers of nurses in New Zealand, covering both the public and private sectors. The data was sought 'as at' a particular day, so that a snapshot picture of the workforce could be obtained.

A second important source of information on the nursing workforce, identified in 1980, was the nurses' Annual Practising Certificates (APC), issued by the Nursing Council. Questions were added to the APC forms to provide data relevant for workforce planning including registration or enrolment status, details about basic nursing qualifications, age, geographical location, type of work and hours worked per week.

Some of the information on the APC renewal forms is provided by nurses on an optional basis; therefore the available data describes a sample rather than the entire workforce. A unique aspect of the data obtained from the APC is the information it provides about nurses who are registered or enrolled but are not currently working as nurses. To date, details from nurses' Annual Practising Certificates still provide the most complete data on the current and latent supply of nurses.

Both the census survey and the APC data had their advantages and disadvantages. The two sources complemented each other and when combined, provided a much more detailed analysis of the supply and potential supply of nurses in New Zealand than was previously available. In 1980, the information obtained from these sources was compiled into a document called 'The Nursing Workforce in New Zealand 1980' (King and Fletcher, 1981).

On the basis of this preliminary data base, some long-held assumptions were questioned. For example, it was apparent that there was, in fact, no overall shortage of nursing staff (as was commonly believed), but the problem lay rather in a maldistribution of nurses over geographical and service areas (King and Fletcher, 1981).

The value of the information held in this 1980 publication led to that data being collected on a regular basis and the Nursing Workforce in New Zealand series has been published every two years since then. These publications have proved particularly valuable for the monitoring of workforce trends that emerge over time.

Another need identified at the 1977 Nursing Manpower Planning Workshop was to collect first-hand information on the worklife of graduate nurses; regarding the various aspects of their length of service, their mobility between different work settings and the nature of the options and plans they had when they decided to leave nursing. A worklife survey of qualified nurses was conducted in 1980 (King and Fletcher, 1980). Findings provided very useful baseline data for nursing management in the employment of part-time staff, and for the development of personnel policies based on the knowledge of the age pattern of the workforce (e.g. expected length of service of graduate nurses and the approximate age of return after child-bearing). It also uncovered the proportion of married nurses in the workforce who had families, many of whom sought different conditions of employment, e.g. part-time work. This contrasted with the late 1960s when married nurses comprised only a very small segment of the practising workforce and were not actively recruited. The pattern of nurses' participation in the workforce has taken on an increasing significance as recent activities and policies focus on issues of staff recruitment and retention.

There have been many other developments in the data collection system since the early 1980s. These have been brought about largely by the need for more timely and more specific data. As new issues in nursing surfaced, procedures for collecting additional data were initiated.

A case in point was a shortage of midwives that became apparent in 1982. Information was needed to formulate a new recruitment policy. Data on the employment of midwives was not collected at that time so six-monthly returns from obstetric/maternity hospitals and units were initiated. The information collected formed the basis for the recruitment policy for midwives and later for a review of training requirements and programmes for their preparation.

Another example, beginning in 1985, was the growing nursing staff shortage in hospitals which prompted a closer monitoring of staffing levels and nursing vacancies. Monthly statistical returns from hospital and area health boards on nursing staffing levels were implemented and monitoring of overseas nurse recruitment was also initiated at this time. The number of overseas nurses who arrived in New Zealand and commenced employment with hospital and area health boards was a crucial piece of information for on-going review of the immigration policy and for co-ordination of the department's overseas recruitment campaign.

A more recent development in our data collection system has arisen out of two identified needs. First, we now require more timely information on the pattern and movement of nurses in the health care system. Secondly, we need to link data on nurses with that of other health professionals, and enlarge our capacity to generate comparative data. This development reflects the changing roles of health professionals and the move towards a transdisciplinary approach in delivering health care.

An integrated information system has been set up which incorporates a wide range of workforce, health service and demographic information. This computerized system takes advantage of the National Payroll System (NPS) through which all hospital and area health board employees are paid. Only aggregate staffing information is extracted from the payroll system. The payroll data base has been further expanded to include information on the sources of recruitment for newly appointed employees and the plans of resigning employees. As issues of recruitment and retention assume more importance this entry and exit data will prove valuable. This information system will have significant impact on national workforce planning as it allows ready access to a comprehensive and accurate data base. It will also permit more detailed analysis of workforce trends and facilitate the forecasting of nursing requirements and supply.

The developing body of knowledge about the nursing workforce has provided the information base required to implement a smooth transfer of nursing education. This forms an objective basis for decision-making and has had a pervasive influence over later workforce policy decisions. Routine procedures have been established for workforce data collection and the improved access to workforce information enables issues to be addressed at the appropriate time rather than after the event. The accumulating historical data base also gives decision-makers the capacity to predict future workforce trends with greater accuracy. More importantly, it facilitated the development of a model to determine future requirements for and supply of nurses.

## Matching requirements and supply

With the initial workforce data base in place, a framework was required to enable the data to be used for analysing the supply and requirement dynamics of the nursing workforce. A model was needed to predict future staffing requirements and to determine appropriate supply through the number of nurses to be trained, retention of nurses in the workforce, and recruitment of nurses from overseas.

In 1982 a group was convened by the Minister of Health, and was designated the Nursing Manpower Planning Committee (NMPC). Members were drawn from a wide background with expertise in nursing and health services management. The Committee's objectives were to develop a tool for nursing workforce planning, to recommend a suitable data collection system and to prepare a national nursing workforce plan. The work of this committee was an important milestone in the development of nursing workforce planning in New Zealand.

In the process of developing a model for projecting requirements, the NMPC used the experience of the Western Interstate Commission on Higher Education (WICHE), Colorado, which had earlier designed a model based on estimating requirements for each category of nurse in a variety of service areas (Gray and Sauer, 1978).

The limitations of the nursing workforce data base at the time the model was being developed required some adaptation of the WICHE model to suit available data. The model was therefore developed to estimate requirements on the basis of 'employment setting' (e.g. public general and obstetric hospital, public psychiatric or psychopaedic hospital, private hospital, public health nursing, etc.) rather than by service area. The predictors used for nurses employed in hospital settings and community settings were nurse to average occupied bed ratios and nurse to population ratios respectively.

A number of assumptions about future trends in demography, health and nursing services were made. Projections were then developed, based on these assumptions and their effect on the predictors. A trend analysis of average occupied beds, nursing staff levels and nurse to average occupied bed ratios (for the previous five to ten years dependent on the availability of data) was used to gauge the effect of the assumptions on the predictors.

In the absence of sufficient historical data, a number of specialist subgroups were set up to provide expert advice and to reach agreement on the range of assumptions adopted. Later, sensitivity analysis to investigate how much a change in each assumption influenced the projected requirements provided a picture of which assumptions were the most critical to future requirements and therefore should be researched most carefully.

Figure 12.2 depicts the supply model adopted (Nursing Manpower Planning Committee, 1985c). The approach taken was to use an aggregate measure of net loss, which summarized factors of retirements, emigration, transfers and movement between active and inactive supply. This was referred to as the 'cohort remainder rate', which was the percentage of the

| Future supply |
|---|

equals

| Current supply minus net loss |
|---|
| (Past      ×     appropriate cohort)<br>(graduates         remainder rate) |

Plus

| Gain from new graduates added during period |
|---|
| (Expected new     cohort remainder)<br>(graduates   ×   rates) |

Plus

| Gain from immigration of overseas graduates during period |
|---|
| (Expected     ×    cohort remainder)<br>(immigrants     rate) |

**Figure 12.2** The supply model.

cohort, or group of nurses graduating during a given period, who remained in the current supply. The 'cohort remainder rate' of the current supply profile could be calculated from the APC data.

Projections of future supply were then obtained by applying the appropriate cohort remainder rate to the cohorts as they 'aged'. Increments to the supply pool of new graduates and immigrants were taken into account and the appropriate cohort remainder rates also applied to these groups.

A baseline supply projection was calculated on the basis of continuation of current policies, and alternative projections explored the effect of policy changes. Sensitivity analysis showed how the model responded to changes in assumptions about future cohort remainder rates, graduate numbers and immigration of overseas nurses. In the process it was found that changes in cohort remainder rates had a more significant effect on the future supply of nurses than alterations to student intakes or immigration policy. This became an important policy consideration and accentuated the need to improve workforce retention.

In 1985 the findings and recommendations of the Nursing Manpower Planning Committee were published in the report 'Nurse Workforce Planning' (Nursing Manpower Planning Committee, 1985d). The requirements and supply model predicted shortages of both registered and enrolled nurses by 1990. Thus the model made it possible to validate the earlier 'guess' on intake numbers made in the absence of a data base. The requirements projection clearly showed this earlier intake estimate to be too low. In anticipation of these shortages, a number of recommendations were made to increase the future supply of qualified nurses and thereby reduce the projected deficit.

The report recommended that measures be taken to increase cohort remainder rates, particularly for younger graduates (Nursing Manpower Planning Committee, 1985a). It was also proposed that the student intakes be increased and that the future levels of these intakes be adjusted according to trends in cohort remainder rates. Revising salaries and other conditions of employment and improving opportunities for professional advancement were also recommended in order to increase retention.

Thus the development of the model and the report had several important effects on nursing policy and initiatives (Nursing Manpower Planning Committee, 1985d). At the government level, they provided substantive data which enabled intake levels of nursing students to be set. The recommendations also resulted in the establishment of an active overseas recruitment and immigration programme. A major review of the preparation and initial employment of nurses was later set up. This will be discussed in more detail later in the chapter. At the local level, the emphasis on the importance of recruitment and retention was taken up by employers and measures to improve these were incorporated into their personnel policies.

*Subsequent developments in matching supply and requirements.* As events unfolded, New Zealand did not have to wait until 1990 to experience a serious shortage of qualified nurses. This shortage occurred in 1985 and urgent measures were implemented to collect data on the actual vacancy levels in order to monitor the situation. The overall vacancy levels in New Zealand public hospitals were as high as 10% for registered nurses, and 11% for enrolled nurses (Department of Health, 1985).

A number of measures were developed to address the actual and projected shortages of nurses.

Restrictions on the entry of overseas nurses to the workforce were relaxed and in 1985 a campaign to actively recruit nurses from the United Kingdom was initiated. Funding support was obtained from the Workforce Development Fund to employ a United Kingdom based liaison person to assist with the recruitment and immigration of British nurses.

Encouraging overseas nurses to work in New Zealand was a satisfactory short-term solution to the shortage problem. An advantage of this strategy was that nurses with specific skills and experience could be recruited for specialist clinical areas where particularly severe shortages were being experienced.

The implications of a continuing shortage had to be taken into account and one longer term solution, considered jointly by the Departments of

Health and Education, was to increase student intakes. A new policy proposal for an increased intake of comprehensive students was approved by the government in 1985 and it was planned to annually increase the student intakes to reach the target level by 1990.

One of the many factors which contributed to the shortage of qualified nurses in 1985–86 was the increased flow of New Zealand nurses to Australia. This could be partly attributed to changes in Australian employment policies for nurses (e.g. reduced working hours and salary increases) and their transfer of nursing education from hospital to tertiary education institutions. The increased emigration highlighted the inter-relationship between New Zealand and Australian labour markets for nurses. A link with nursing workforce planners in Australia had since been established to share workforce information and planning expertise so that in future, overseas events can be taken into account in our workforce planning.

The nursing shortage became an industrial issue and was used effectively in salary negotiations resulting in substantial salary increases for nurses in 1985.

Since 1985, marked improvements have been noted in the cohort remainder rates and in vacancy levels which we continue to monitor. Vacancy levels for registered nurses have decreased from the 10% high in 1985 to about 4%, and this has now stabilized.

The need to review and revise the requirements and supply projections regularly was recognized. The first review of the assumptions underlying the requirements projections was carried out in May 1987.

There were two major outcomes from this review. First, new requirements projections, like those calculated in 1985, predicted a continual growth in the requirements for registered nurses. Secondly, it was recommended that the requirements model should be further developed and an alternative predictor to 'nurse to average occupied bed ratios' be found. A new predictor was needed in response to the increasing utilization of outpatient and community services and higher patient turnover. These predicted trends could not be adequately reflected in average occupied bed numbers.

The models defined the critical supply and requirement factors of the nursing workforce. The interaction between what were traditionally thought of as quantitative factors (for example attrition rates) and qualitative factors (for example job satisfaction, management and career structures, quality assurance, etc.) was emphasized. The process of sensitivity analysis enabled priorities for policy measures and further research to be established. The need to retain qualified nurses in the workforce was identified as a top priority.

Thus the requirements and supply models provided an important framework for nursing workforce planning activities. The models yielded projections for future requirements and supply of qualified nurses in New

Zealand, and pointed to a likely mismatch between the two. In particular, it was the predicted undersupply of qualified nurses in the 1985 report which had a direct and major impact on policies and initiatives relating to student intakes, immigration levels and retention measures (Nursing Manpower Planning Committee, 1985b).

## Recruitment and retention studies relating to nursing service

As the transfer of nursing education progressed, nursing services were increasingly provided by a predominantly qualified nursing workforce. The focus of workforce planning gradually shifted from nursing education to nursing service issues.

The impact of the cohort remainder rates as a major factor in the supply of nurses and the prevailing nursing shortage in 1985, reaffirmed the priority to improve workforce recruitment and retention. Numerous studies on the subject have been undertaken. Staff retention problems were addressed by research into job satisfaction among nurses. The implications for nursing management structures of a largely qualified workforce were noted. This is especially relevant with the increasing number of comprehensive graduates commencing their nursing practice. A major review into the preparation and initial employment of nurses was finally set up in 1986. Other studies into the needs of comprehensive students and the facilitation of their transition from students to beginning practitioners were undertaken.

The causes of workforce attrition are varied and complex. The lack of job satisfaction has been noted as a particularly common reason for staff turnover (Mottaz, 1988). Currently a major study of this issue is being carried out in New Zealand (Ng, Cram and Jenkins, 1988). It involves a longitudinal survey of a sample of nurses over a period of four months to track the decision making path of nurses who have resigned or who have remained during that time. Personal factors and job characteristics that lead to attrition and retention can then be identified. A follow-up study is also planned to identify particular centres of nursing excellence. Overall, the study aims to identify measures to reduce workforce attrition and to provide guidelines for administrative and staff development initiatives to attract qualified ex-employees back into the workforce.

The changing pattern of staffing towards greater numbers of qualified staff had major implications for nursing management structures. Previously these were based on the need to ensure the safety and competence of a largely unqualified workforce through close supervision and controlled work practices. They were not suitable for a largely qualified and professional workforce that was educated to make autonomous decisions on patient care. The slow move to adopt primary nursing is still an issue for nursing in New Zealand. Both issues have potentially adverse effects on nursing job satisfaction.

As the first comprehensive graduates began to enter the workforce some of these problems emerged. Miller's study in 1978 was one of the first to document the experience of the early comprehensive graduates as they commenced practice. The bureaucratic structure of hospitals and communication systems in particular were perceived by comprehensive graduates as preventing them from functioning as professionals (Miller, 1978).

Overall, the transition of nursing education progressed very smoothly. However, by 1986 there were emerging concerns such as the real reasons behind prevailing nursing shortage and the need to address issues related to the initial practice of new graduates. It was timely to re-examine aspects of both nursing education and service. The Review of the Preparation and Initial Employment of Nurses (RPIEN) was set up. Its format was a broad consultative one. Submissions were widely sought and a workshop was held to review the issues and develop strategies for future action. The workshop group comprised invited participants from a variety of backgrounds representing consumers, nursing service, nursing management, nursing education and other health professionals.

This review put forward a list of proposals for action. On the issue of initial employment of new comprehensive graduates, it recommended major improvements to induction and orientation programmes for new graduate employees. Other recommendations included facilitation of recruitment and retention of new graduates in specific service areas, and reappraisal of nurses' working environment including nursing structures, management and conditions of employment. The need to strengthen communication between nursing service and nursing education based on mutually accepted goals for the preparation of nurses for the health services in New Zealand, was also identified. Awareness of the increasing relevance of the social and cultural context of nursing practice was reflected in recommendations which emphasized a bicultural approach to nursing education and service (Department of Health, 1986h). Subsequently, the Department of Health supported the National Council of Maori Nurses to hold a national hui (gathering) to discuss the views of Maori people on nursing and health related matters. There is an on-going commitment to improve recruitment and retention of Maori people into nursing and to foster Maori cultural values in the health care system.

The importance of the adjustment of comprehensive graduates to the workplace and the facilitation of their transition from students to practitioners has since received much recognition. Other research into the initial practice of comprehensive graduates has also attracted funding support from the Department of Health through its Workforce Development Fund.

The difficulties experienced by new comprehensive graduates were pinpointed in a study by Wootton in 1987. The study sought to identify factors which aid or hinder the transition from student to practising nurse. Specific suggestions were made which involved actions on the part of both employers and educational institutions. These included planned orientation, e.g. preceptorship schemes, support networks for comprehensive graduates; clear identification of the expectations of the new staff nurse; clarification of the role of the staff nurse and of the enrolled nurse; and better planned clinical elective experience for third year students. Knowledge and skills aside, the study also highlighted the importance of attitudes in the adjustment process. This referred to the attitudes of both graduates and those in the work environment. Receptive and welcoming attitudes on the part of other staff towards the new graduates could help ease the transition from students to practitioners.

The experience of third-year students during their clinical electives and their future employment plans were surveyed by Perry in 1987. It was noted that students in this study rated personal development factors as more important for achieving personal satisfaction in nursing than either work conditions or professional development. This finding contributed another dimension to the understanding of nursing job satisfaction. In general these students rated themselves as competent in most areas of nursing practice at a beginning practitioner level.

The findings of these studies helped stimulate initiatives to improve nursing management. Management workshops, which received funding from the Workforce Development Fund, were held throughout New Zealand for nurse managers. Hospitals had also begun to make provision for improved orientation programmes to cater for the needs of new graduate nurses. Meantime, attempts to alleviate nursing shortages and improve workforce retention had been initiated. Some examples of these included the provision of funding for refresher courses to attract nurses back into the workforce and short courses to improve skills in the clinical areas with recruitment difficulties.

Recruitment and retention of the nursing workforce remains an ongoing issue for management and for workforce planning. The challenge is to provide job and career satisfaction in a workforce largely comprising qualified nurses with expectations of professional autonomy. Recognition of their need to be able to practise according to their preparation, and to have scope for innovation and incentives for advancement based upon their nursing practice, is important (Shaw, 1986).

## Current developments: an increasing emphasis on qualitative aspects of nursing workforce planning

The early data collected was primarily quantitative. It provided information on the nature of the workforce: its size and composition; distribution by employment and practice settings and type of preparation and registration. It also provided a profile of nurses in the New Zealand workforce: age, sex and geographical distribution.

The transfer of nursing education and the accompanying transition to a qualified nursing workforce, highlighted the need for more qualitative information for planning efficient nursing services. At the same time, the changes of society have affected the requirements of health care delivery systems and, thus, of nursing care.

The first national attempt to determine the level and mix of nursing staff needed in the different settings were made in 1980. Nine working parties were set up to define the role of the nurse in specific functional areas of practice; to define the categories of nurse required and to prepare guidelines for health agencies to assist them in preparing a workforce plan for each functional area (Department of Health, 1982). An extensive trial of these guidelines however found them to be unsatisfactory for identifying requirements and it was recommended that they not be adopted (Department of Health, 1983). These guidelines were untimely as the staffing requirements calculated were based on a qualified nurse workforce at a time when many hospitals were still using student nurses to provide services. There was also a wide variation in how they were applied by different hospital boards, which greatly limited their usefulness for national planning. Although the guidelines were not adopted, the process had an important bearing on the future direction of workforce planning on a nationnal basis. They confirmed the need to re-examine the role of national workforce planning in relation to the role of planning at the local level.

The existing planning model for projecting nursing requirements focuses on identifying relevant measures of workload indicators based on level of service throughput. In response to the wider health service trends of increasing emphasis on community care and primary health care, the roles of nurses have diversified and broadened. Changing social, educational, cultural, economic and demographic conditions also influence patterns of nursing practice. The Review of Preparation and Initial Employment of Nurses (RPIEN) recommended that the scope and functions of nurses be redefined, and the appropriate level and mix of nurses in different settings be reviewed (Department of Health, 1986a). The latter would ensure provision of high quality nursing care which is cost-effective.

A group was set up to redefine the scope and function of nursing in New Zealand in 1987. This involved several steps. First, the issues in New Zealand society and the relevant changes in the health services which might affect the scope and function of nursing currently and in the future were identified. After this the elements of the function of nursing were identified and used as a basis for identifying the parameters to which nursing could expand. The resulting statements of belief on the scope and function of nursing were published and widely distributed in April 1988 (National Action Group, 1988). This document is expected to provide a basis for the on-going development of nursing as a profession; for nursing education and for nursing workforce planning.

The Health Department, through the Workforce Development Fund, is currently planning a research project to look at nursing and the competencies required at different levels and settings. This will provide information leading to an assessment of the appropriate level and mix of nursing staff in each setting.

It is becoming apparent that planning needs to recognize the other external factors which impact on the nursing workforce in the broader political, social and economic context. The planning model is currently under review to incorporate a broader dimension which takes this multitude of factors into account. The extent to which nursing is effectively meeting the needs of the health service also has to be addressed.

## CONCLUSION

This chapter has developed a discussion on the impact of research in shaping policy decisions related to the nursing workforce. Several distinct issues have been identified which serve to illustrate the role of research.

The initiative for the transfer of nursing education from hospital-based training to the general system of education arose out of a variety of considerations. A major impetus came from early studies in the 1960s on student attrition from hospital programmes. Findings of high student wastage first prompted a review of the nursing education system which culminated in the transfer.

Research had a continuing input into the actual implementation of the transfer. In order to determine intake levels and the pace of transfer, formal procedures were initiated to gather relevant workforce data. A profile of the nursing workforce was also developed from the data base which allowed for a quantitative assessment of the nature of the workforce. Overall this data base facilitated a structured, analytical approach to policy making.

The development of a planning model marked the next phase of workforce studies and provided a framework for analysing the balance between supply and requirements of the nursing workforce. Projections on future requirements and supply for the nursing workforce had a direct bearing on policies relating to student intake levels and overseas recruitment. In particular, the powerful impact of cohort remainder rates on the size of the practising workforce was singled out by the model.

Issues of recruitment and retention of the workforce therefore became a major concern. Job satisfaction studies were initiated. Problems also arose with the emergence of a largely qualified workforce. Changes to nursing management were required to enable nurses to practise professionally and to enhance job satisfaction. Of particular concern was the initial practice of new comprehensive graduates as they began to enter the workforce. Studies in this area emphasized the importance of orientation and induction programmes to facilitate the students' transition to practitioners. The Review of Preparation and Initial Employment of Nurses (RPIEN) was especially instrumental in addressing these issues and effecting changes.

The present focus of research is on qualitative workforce planning issues. Two of the recommendations from RPIEN relating to this have been followed up. These involve redefining the scope and function of nursing, and reviewing the appropriate level and mix of nursing staff in different practice settings.

Currently in New Zealand there is a plethora of reports and reviews into a wide range of areas covering health services, accident compensation schemes, education, and the whole framework of social policy. These will effect changes to the health services. There is a clear need to examine and research these external factors as they impinge on the nursing workforce.

In conclusion, it is important to reinforce the strategic relevance of research to planning. In our experience, research has facilitated a comprehensive and co-ordinated approach to policy formulation over time. However, one must also be mindful of the long lead time involved, both in the process of workforce planning and in effecting policy initiatives. As a consequence of this long lead time, the impact of research on policies may be less explicit in some cases. It is a persistent challenge for research to target the information requirements of decision-makers so that research findings can be translated into useful and timely policy action. The importance of the Department of Health's commitment to take a leading role in the development of the workforce, and to adopt an appropriate organizational structure which facilitates the integration of research and policy, cannot be understated. On the basis of New Zealand's experience, nursing workforce planning and research have had a significant role to play in policy development and, through this, have directed major change in New Zealand nursing.

## REFERENCES

Carpenter, H. (1971) *An improved system of nursing education for New Zealand*, Department of Health, Wellington, pp. 5–7.

Department of Education (1972) *Nursing education in New Zealand*, Wellington, p. 22.

Department of Health (1979) Management Services and Research Unit in collaboration with the Division of Nursing, *Nursing staff employed by hospital boards in New Zealand 1977 and 1979 compared*, Occasional paper, no. 10, Wellington.

Department of Health (1982) 'Report of nine nursing manpower planning working parties', unpublished, Wellington.

Department of Health (1983) 'Report on the testing of the nursing manpower planning guidelines', unpublished, Wellington.

Department of Health (1985) unpublished statistics, Wellington.

Department of Health (1986a) *Preparation and initial employment*, Wellington, pp. 39–40.

Department of Health (1986b) *Preparation and initial employment*, Wellington, p. 86.

Department of Health (1986c) *Preparation and initial employment*, Wellington, p. 87.

Department of Health (1986d) *Preparation and initial employment*, p. 87.

Department of Health (1986e) *Preparation and initial employment*, Wellington, p. 87.

Department of Health (1986f) *Review of the preparation and initial employment of nurses*, Wellington, p. 88.

Department of Health (1986g) *Preparation and initial employment*, Wellington, p. 88.

Department of Health (1986h) *Preparation and initial employment*, Wellington, pp. 68–69.

Department of Health (1987a) unpublished statistics, Wellington.

Department of Health (1987b) unpublished statistics, Wellington.

Department of Statistics (1988a) *Official Yearbook 1987–88*, Government Printer, Wellington, p. 128.

Department of Statistics (1988b) *Official Yearbook 1987–1988*, Government Printer, Wellington.

Department of Statistics (1988c) *Official Yearbook 1987–88*, Government Printer, Wellington, p. 213.

Gray, R. and Sauer, K. (1978) *Nursing resources and requirements: a guide for state-level planning*, Western Interstate Commission on Higher Education, Boulder, Colorado.

King, B.E. and Fletcher, M.P. (1980) *The work-life of qualified nurses in one metropolitan hospital: a pilot project*, Special Report Series no. 57, Management Services and Research Unit, Department of Health, Wellington.

King, B.E. and Fletcher, M.P. (1981) *The nursing workforce in New Zealand 1980*, Management Services and Research Unit, Department of Health, Wellington.

Miller, N.R. (1978) 'The problems experienced by graduates of student based comprehensive nursing programmes as they provide nursing care in general hospitals', unpublished Masters dissertation, University of Auckland.

Mottaz, C.J. (1988) Work satisfaction among hospital nurses, *Hospital and Health Services Administration*, vol. 33, no. 1 pp. 57–74.

National Action Group (1988) *Review of the preparation and initial employment of nurses, statement from the workshop on the scope and function of nursing*, National Action Group Publication, no. 1, Wellington.

New Zealand Nursing Education and Research Foundation (1977) *New Zealand nursing manpower planning report*, NERF Studies in Nursing: no. 4, Wellington, p. 11.

New Zealand Statute (1971) *Nurses Act 1971*, no. 78, s. 3, Wellington.

Ng, S.H., Cram, F. and Jenkins, L. (1988) 'Job satisfaction and job withdrawal among staff nurses in public hospitals: a longitudinal study', unpublished, University of Otago.

Nursing Manpower Planning Committee (1985a) *Nurse Workforce planning*, p. 17.

Nursing Manpower Planning Committee (1985b) *Nurse workforce planning*, p. 20.

Nursing Manpower Planning Committee (1985c) *Nurse workforce planning*, Department of Health, Wellington, p. 60.

Nursing Manpower Planning Committee (1985d) *Nurse workforce planning*, 78 pp.

Perry, J. (1987) *Transition from student to graduate: phase one, profile of third year comprehensive nursing students*, Department of Nursing Studies, Massey University.

Shaw, S. (1986) 'Another time, another challenge' in *Horizons of care: papers presented at Norman Peryer Forum, 6–8 December, 1985.* Nursing Education and Research Foundation, Wellington.

Wootton, R.M. *Orientation of the newly registered comprehensive nurse for work in the health services. A study of the transition from student to employee and practising nurse in one large hospital board*, Department of Nursing Studies, Christchurch Polytechnic, pp. 34–36.

# CHAPTER THIRTEEN

# Research as a modifier of the constraints in developing nursing practice in South Africa: an overview

*Charlotte Searle*

## INTRODUCTION

Prior to World War II low levels of industrial development, urbanization, communication and educational networks, national and *per capita* incomes characterized the South African social situation. Centres of industrial, commercial and educational excellence existed only in the metropolitan areas. The health services were modelled on the public health philosophy and local authority and voluntary hospital systems characteristic of the pre-World War II approach in Britain. Nursing philosophy, nursing management approaches and nursing education were deeply rooted in the British system from which they originated. Answers to the innumerable problems besetting nursing in South Africa were sought in Britain.

As a result of the great economic depression of the 1930s all social services, both state and voluntary, were not able to meet the clamant needs of the population.

The nursing system failed to meet the nation's needs for nurses because of archaic management concepts and because the nursing education system was based on the hospital-nursing school model. 'The probationers' comprised the main workforce in the hospital. Nursing education was merely a casual by-product of the hospital system. The long hours of work in the name of 'education', the mere pittances in monthly allowances, the poor standards of accommodation for students, the lack of inservice education and further education opportunities for nurses, the inadequate opportunities for career advancement, the 'handmaiden to the doctor' image that many nurses presented, the inadequate, understaffed, service-dominated educational system which resulted in a continuous state of 'undeclared war' between nurse educators and nurse administrators, had all contributed to the low self-image as well as poor public image of the nursing profession. All this had virtually brought the profession to its knees.

As a then British Dominion, South Africa entered World War II in 1939 with an inadequate, overworked and overextended nursing service. In the years between 1939 and 1945 all its resources were directed to the war effort. As a result of the war needs of Britain and the Allied Forces, industrialization and urbanization developed very rapidly. Internal population shifts and influx of people from across the national borders, as well as large numbers of sick and wounded British and Allied soldiers who were diverted to South Africa to regain their health, brought the health services to near collapse. The nursing profession being the main provider of health care personnel bore the brunt of this rapid social and demographic change. Inevitably standards of care deteriorated and gross dissatisfaction occurred in the ranks of the profession.

With few exceptions neither the health care authorities nor the medical profession, at that stage, saw the nurse as a colleague of the doctor. She was there to carry out the orders of doctors and of the health care authorities. No thought was given to the fact that nurses might find answers to the many ills plaguing the health services, and the nursing profession in particular.

## THE STATUS OF NURSES

By the end of World War II the nursing profession in South Africa vigorously asserted itself by convincing Parliament that the time had come to separate the control of the medical, nursing and pharmacy professions by establishing separate statutory Councils for peer group control of each of these professions, giving these Councils an equal status in law and the three professions an equal *de jure* status. The *de facto* status had to be earned. The concept of equal status was further strengthened by providing for reciprocal representation between the medical and dental and nursing councils to strengthen the concept of equality and collegiality. This concept was later extended to the Pharmacy Council (Medical Act 1944, The Pharmacy Act 1944 and the Nursing Act 1944). For half a century the organized profession had, with limited success, made representations to the national health care authorities about diverse nursing matters. By 1942 a new generation of nurse leaders decided to undertake 'action research' and to use the scientific method to study the problems of the profession, to prepare memoranda presenting their case and to recommend solutions based on careful identification of relevant data, sound analysis and deductions (SA Trained Nurses' Association, 1943a).

This memorandum which was based on careful research made a major impact on the perception which Parliament, the health care authorities and the medical profession had of the nursing profession in South Africa. A willingness to listen, to debate, to identify social and economic restraints that would slow down implementation of much needed change, emerged. Interim compromises and solutions were agreed upon between the Minister and the Governing Board of the SA Trained Nurses' Association. These were the immediate effects of action based on the scientific method of study of the problems of the nursing profession. The then Minister of Welfare and Demobilization, Advocate Harry Lawrence, stated to the delegation presenting the memorandum

'the nurses have presented their case in a carefully researched scientific manner which makes each argument indisputable. They have laid an unassailable foundation for the future of their profession as a major health profession in this country. No other health profession has stated its case so succinctly, so logically and with such accuracy as to its proven importance in the life of the nation, its potential if that which impedes its growth and development is removed, and its confidence and pride in that which it has achieved and plans to implement. The nursing profession is a profession that must control its own destiny and must legally be placed on an equal footing with that of the medical, dental and pharmacy professions. I will ensure that this is done by making the Nursing Bill a Government Bill, I will see that the first Nursing Council is established during my term of office. Your responsible, professional, scholarly and clearly scientific approach has earned this recognition of your profession' (SA Trained Nurses' Association, 1943b).

## FUTURE DEVELOPMENT

The success of this approach to the Minister convinced the participants in this interview that the nursing profession in South Africa could only redress the many weaknesses in its system by systematic research into the diverse ills that beset the profession. At that stage the leaders identified some areas which most urgently needed research, namely issues relating to:

student nurse recruitment, selection and attrition;
nursing education with emphasis on nursing education systems and methods, introduction of experimental schemes, nurse educator preparation, success rates in the national examinations, curriculum content, and resolution of conflicts between education and service needs;
nursing service with emphasis on the socio-economic status of nurses,

work studies, the role and functions of the nurse administrator and cost containment in hospitals.

The consensus at that stage was that the quality of nursing care would improve once the more blatant shortcomings in the whole nursing system were eliminated. Medical practice which had undergone tremendous growth and development in the war years and which was ushering in a period of unprecedented scientific and technological development would change health care so dramatically that nursing would have to develop new approaches to provide scientific humane nursing care. This would need scientific study of the implications for nursing. This was a largely unknown challenge, so clinical nursing research was not considered opportune at that stage. However, they clearly subscribed to the concept that 'the scientific efforts of the doctors to cure or heal must be supplemented by the intelligent efforts of the nurse to apply the remedies prescribed in the best possible manner' (Fenwick, 1889). Clinical research had to come but the parlous state of the nursing profession resulted in an obsession among nurse leaders for research into the problems that prevented growth and development in the profession. Research into the quality of care and into new approaches to clinical care were relegated to the future. The leaders of the profession clearly believed that good clinical practice was dependent on improvement in the entire structure and status of the nursing profession. By 1947 the profession was geared to accept the challenges of the post-war period.

A sign of the greatness of the older leaders who were all products of hospital-based diploma courses was that the young university graduate in their midst was not only given a hearing but was actively encouraged to further studies so that she could ultimately build up a cadre of nurse researchers who had the necessary university education, and who had the ability to collaborate with researchers in other disciplines, particularly in the social sciences and with researchers in medicine in the clinical field. These leaders were adamant that nursing must identify its extensive body of knowledge and must augment this knowledge through research so that a firm scientific basis of practice could be developed. They urged this young graduate in their midst to undertake further study so that she may assimilate the principles and methods of research of other disciplines for adaptation to nursing research. This approach is not unique to nursing's development of its research potential. All modern research in the medical, biological, physical, geophysical, chemical, aerospace and indeed social science arenas require tremendous co-operation by numbers of scientists in related fields and have developed in this way. The faith of the leaders was impregnable but the way to achievement of the ideal was a long and arduous one.

## THE NECESSITY FOR RESEARCH

Research in nursing could only be developed if the profession as a whole accepted the need for research and if selected members were willing to undergo the rigorous educational process that is basic to the development of research skills. Brotherston, speaking at a conference on the planning of nursing studies at Sevres, stated that 'whereas the ability and the opportunity to carry out research must be limited to a minority in any profession, an urgent and understanding sense of the need for research should be a part of the mental equipment of every member of any profession worthy of the name' (Brotherston, 1960).

This understanding and sense of need was absent among the majority of the members of the nursing profession in the pre- and early post-World War II periods. This was mainly due to the fact that at that stage university education in nursing studies was limited to the preparation of nurse educators at three universities by means of a one-year post-registration diploma course. Preparation for the inculcation of research attitudes and guidance in research principles and methodology were absent from these courses.

The negative attitude of the doctors towards nursing research fostered a sense of negativism.

Nursing degrees were not available at South African, or British universities at that stage. The first nurse in South Africa to obtain a master's degree (1951) did so in Sociology. She subsequently obtained a Doctor of Philosophy in the same discipline (1964). It is ironic that this nurse was unable to obtain any form of financial support for the research component of the master's degree or for the research for the thesis for the doctorate, because all the authorities who were approached were unable to accept that a nurse could do quality research despite the evidence of a well-prepared research proposal. In all cases the advisers to these authorities were medical doctors from the academic field. However, the results of the research for these two degrees had a profound effect on nursing and nursing education in South Africa.

## RESEARCH AND NURSING PRACTICE

The first study 'The problem of the shortage of nursing personnel in Transvaal Public Hospitals', was augmented by a series of unpublished 'operational research' studies in the hospitals of that province (Searle, 1951). The study and its follow-up studies into specific aspects of the problem had a revolutionary effect on the organization of the nursing services, management practices, the socio-economic status of the nurse and the nursing education system in the province. Through the efforts of the Hospitals and Health Services Co-ordinating Council of the Union of

South Africa, and of the South African Nursing Association, extensive improvements were also implemented by the national health department, the other provincial health authorities and by local authorities. This was possible because the responsible officers, particularly the officers of the Public Service Commission, the Directors of Nursing Services in the various provinces, the Chief Administrative Officers in these services and the members of the Board of the South African Nursing Association studied the research findings, saw the merit in the data obtained and in the recommendations and gave the reform process their full support.

## NURSE RESEARCHERS

Because resistance to the establishment of nursing degrees was strong, even in the ranks of nurses and parliamentarians it was not possible to establish the first nursing degree course in South Africa until 1956. It took two decades to take nursing education into the rest of the South African universities. The result was that the first masters' and doctoral programmes could not be established until 1967.

The development of the research component of the nursing degrees was hampered by the lack of nursing faculty with sound preparation in nursing research, for at this stage the few senior nurse educators who held degrees did so at baccalaureate level in the social sciences or in the liberal arts. Sadly the few nurses who had qualified as medical practitioners were not interested in assisting the profession with this particular phase of its development. A further constraint was the lack of suitable publications for publishing nursing research. The result was that research that was done had either to be published in book form or in pamphlet or bound, typed copy form. This restricted the distribution of South African nursing research. Nurses had yet to progress to publication of research registers and research journals.

The ever-present shortage of funds for nursing research was also a powerful inhibiting factor. Those who held the purse strings for research funds had yet to satisfy themselves that nursing as a discipline justified the expenditure of scarce research funds. To counter these constraints and with an unshakeable faith in the need for research to provide the knowledge base for further developments in nursing, the leaders of the profession set themselves the task to prove the importance of nursing research for the development of the health services, and began to lay the foundation for the development of research attitudes and research skills at a variety of levels in nursing. The aim was to awaken an awareness among the current and future nurse leaders of the importance of research for nursing management, education and practice.

The President of the SA Nursing Council, Miss C A Nothard RRC clinched an argument for the need for nursing research by stating 'Nursing progress without research is a house without a foundation' (Nothard, 1951).

## THE INTRODUCTORY APPROACH

As it was recognized that the preparation of nurse researchers with masters and doctoral degrees would take a considerable time, steps were taken to include research courses in all diploma courses offered at post-registration level to nurses holding three-year nursing diplomas. These courses were given at universities or at nursing colleges. This was one of the most positive steps taken by the nurse leaders, for it produced a cadre of senior nurses who possessed the right attitude to research in nursing, who had a measure of research knowledge and skills, who could read research reports with insight and who were prepared to co-operate in the development of higher degrees for nurses where the research skills could be developed. In particular they were willing to co-operate in research programmes initiated by the new breed of nurse, the university graduate. What was even more important was the fact that they were ready, where relevant, to implement the research findings into their respective organizations. This introductory approach laid the real foundation for nursing research in South Africa between 1951 and 1960. In the process a surprisingly large amount of valuable research was done, and what is so important, was utilized in the development of the diverse aspects of nursing. It has been possible to identify 74 studies undertaken by students on post-registration diploma courses which have made a marked and lasting contribution to the development of nursing practice in South Africa. This research dealt with such issues as:

organization and management of nursing services
the system of nursing education
nursing curricula and didactics
nursing ethics
hospital management, planning, equipment, services, supplies and communication systems
role definitions, evaluation of post structures, recruitment of nurses
personnel management; cultural issues in nursing
nursing techniques and practices and inter professional relationships (National Nursing Research Register, Vol. I, 1984.)

The thrust of the statement that this introductory approach to nursing research had a profound effect on nursing practice lies in the fact that these were not nurses holding degrees who made this important contribution to the development of their profession. They were persons holding a three-year diploma from a hospital nursing school who had been given additional education with a significant component of research methodology. These studies can be described as descriptive studies utilizing the scientific method for identification and solving of problems. It is this type of research approach that should be taught to all nurses in nursing diploma programmes for it leads to reasoned thinking, establishment of facts, logical means of searching for solutions and careful drawing of conclusions. It is the beginning of a research-minded approach to nursing practice for the nurse who has not had the benefit of a degree education in nursing. By the time nurses with masters and doctoral degrees became available to the profession, an elementary research foundation had been laid, and the findings of the research process had begun to whittle away at traditionalism and the tendency to reproduce the solutions operative in other countries to assuage the ills of nursing practice in South Africa. These 'beginner' researchers have now had their work listed in the National Nursing Research Register Vol. I, 1984.

## THE RECOGNITION OF NURSING RESEARCH

When the thesis of the first nurse to obtain a Doctor of Philosophy in South Africa (1964) was acclaimed by the History Society of South Africa and by the Medical History Society of South Africa as research which must be classified as Africana of outstanding worth, nursing research in South Africa took its place alongside the research of other related disciplines (Searle, 1965). Health authorities, the medical profession, the educational authorities, the community in general, and in particular the nursing profession now saw nursing in a new light, namely that of nation builder. The profession and its role and functions took on new meaning and dimensions. It was suddenly realized that the nursing profession is a powerful force in the health services of this country and in the social development of the many different peoples constituting the nation. Nursing research was established and had earned 'house room' in the research systems of this country.

Research provided the basis for the development of the profession at all levels. It determined the nature and extent of the practice of nursing, its input into the development of the health services and identified its strengths and weaknesses.

## NURSING RESEARCH AS BASIS FOR PRACTICE

The research of masters and doctoral students in nursing, and of other contemporary nurse researchers have had a profound effect on nursing practice and on the development of the profession. The quality of this work has led to extensive implementation of the findings in the diverse practice situations. This has resulted in many radical role changes, new approaches to old problems, a new professional image in many fields of practice and a new level of confidence in the way the practitioner plays her role (National

Nursing Research Registers, Vol. I (1984), Vol. II (1985), Vol. III (1986), Vol. IV (1987), Vol. V (1988). Improvement in the care of patients, in personnel satisfaction in stress-ridden areas and in student nurse education are the main off-spins of this research.

In the ever-changing kaleidoscope of nursing practice, on-going research is necessary. This is now accepted by health care authorities and by the authorities controlling research funds. Nurses are now obtaining their fair share of research funds from their universities, the Medical Research Council, the Human Sciences Research Council and a number of Trusts sponsoring research grants. It is acknowledged that research is changing the practice of nursing to enable it to meet the demands of the incoming century. This in itself is testimony to the work done by nurse researchers in this country. In addition, a nurse is a member of the assessment panel for research grants made available to nurses by the Human Sciences Research Council. The majority of Trusts which sponsor research projects have a nurse on the panel when assessing applications from nurses for research funds.

It is significant that between 1951 and 1984 a total of 344 nursing studies were recognized as being suitable for inclusion in Vol. I of the National Nursing Research Register. In 1985 a total of 111 were accepted for listing in Vol. II of the register. In 1986 (Vol. III) the number was 141, in 1987 (Vol. IV) it was 138, and in 1988 (Vol. V) it was 184. Approximately 50% of the research now being done is in the clinical field. Doctors in academic hositals are now regularly commenting on the high standard of clinical research done by nurses.

The work reflected in the registers does not include the large number of small descriptive studies undertaken in the work situation, neither does it include the type of systematic scientific study which results in publication of a series of guidelines for practise known as 'The Brief Series'. It also does not include the extensive research undertaken by lecturers for the preparation of teaching material which take the form of books or study guides. These books and study guides are making a profound impact on the education of nurses (and hence the practice) not only in South Africa but in many parts of Africa where the language medium in the professional nursing schools is English. Learning leads to improvement in practise, and for this reason such publications are researched meticulously. Research which resulted in two publications – *Professional Practice: A South African Perspective* (Searle, 1986) and *Ethos of Nursing and Midwifery – a general perspective* (Searle, 1987) have made a major impact on the professional nursing practice in South Africa. The delineation of the scope of practice of nurses and midwives within an evolving health care and political situation and the clear delineation of the legal and ethical situation governing nursing in South Africa ensures that the nursing profession retains its status as equal partner with the medical profession and as the key provider of health care in this country. This research is widely used by health care authorities, the nursing and legal professions. There is evidence that doctors are making a close study of these works for they realize that they have lost their handmaidens but have gained an indispensable professional partner. They are still recovering from the shock that research has revealed that the South African law and the provisions of the Nursing Act places the dependent function of the nurse on the law and not on the doctor and provides for the nurse to have an interdependent function with the doctor and other health workers, as well as an independent function. The fact that research has shown that the patient is legally the patient of the doctor, as well as of the nurse in charge, and that the nurse is accountable for his/her own *actions* but is required in the interest of patient care to co-operate on a collegial basis with the patient's doctor and other members of the health team, came as a profound shock to the medical profession and to health care providers. The doctors always believed that they had sole rights to the patient care situation (Searle, 1986).

## BROAD SPECTRUM OF NURSING RESEARCH

Nursing research now covers a wide spectrum of issues. Nursing research in South Africa can now be classified into research relating to all the diverse aspects of nursing education, nursing administration, fields of employment for nurses, provision of health care facilities, professional development, communication, professional relationship issues, community services, primary health care development, improvement in clinical practice for both acute and chronic sickness in all phases of man's life, provision of nursing care in the formidable communicable diseases such as the deadly haemor-rhagic diseases (Lassa fever, Ebola, Marburg's disease and Congo–Crimean haemorrhagic fever). Aids is now being added to the problem diseases requiring meticulous research for safe compassionate nursing practice.

Research in the field of theory and model development is in its infancy but is making steady progress. A major thrust in nursing research is now directed to clinical nursing research, embracing in particular the preven-tative, promotive, curative and rehabilitative aspects of health care throughout man's life span. Particular emphasis is being placed on research into the value of patient education and the development of high quality care in all aspects of nursing. Due to the paucity of suitable literature for the South African scene with its multiplicity of languages and cultures marked attention is also being given to research in acute nursing (crisis nursing) in a range of some 25 health care specialties with intent to publish nursing literature which could be readily available to the profession. This is a continuous, if slow, process. Historical research and research in the soci-ology of nursing is on-going and is aimed at ensuring that the nurse knows who and what she is and what are the main trends in nursing and in the social conditions for which she must gear her professional development.

## CONCLUSION

Nursing research is the main modifier of the constraints in developing nursing practice in South Africa. It is accepted as such by the nursing profession, by the health care authorities and by the authorities financing research from private and/or public funds. It is the main determinant of whether the nursing profession in South Africa will measure up to the demands society is making on it, demands which will accelerate as the population explosion grows apace and as the changing social and political situation makes its impact felt on all walks of life. Nursing research has proved its indispensability as a determinant for nursing practice. It now has to provide direction for coping with the demands of the twenty-first century.

In the process towards maturity it has helped to evolve a South African philosophy of nursing, and a system of nursing service, nursing education and clinical practice which is relevant to the needs of a country which is both a Developed and Developing Country in Africa. It has:

- placed the nursing profession on a par with the medical, dental and pharmacy professions;
- placed the nurse administrator in a position of power within the health care hierarchy;
- extended the scope of practice of nurses in an open-ended manner to the extent that the nursing profession is now recognized as the main provider of health care in South Africa;
- evolved a system of nursing education which places it squarely in the tertiary education system with professional nursing education being available only at universities or at colleges of nursing in association with universities. The phasing out of all hospital-based nursing schools will be completed by 1990. All professional nursing education is of 4 years duration and is comprehensive to meet the health needs of the South African nation. All nurses qualify in general, psychiatric and community nursing and in midwifery. Specialization in these disciplines, or in aspects thereof, follow on the basic registration either through post-registration diplomas or post-graduate degrees. Nurse educators have been placed on an equal footing with other educators in the tertiary education system;
- developed clinical nursing practice into an open-ended scientific discipline with the quality of care the dominant feature.

The professional 'house of nursing' has laid a firm foundation for itself, by development of research relevant to its needs.

## REFERENCES

*N.B.* Due to the number of research publications scrutinized it is not possible, for want of space, to list all the publications. The volume of research registers, year and code numbers of the research are listed to facilitate further reference.

Brotherston, J.H.F. (1960) Research-mindedness and the health professions, in *Learning to Investigate Nursing Problems.* International Council of Nurses and Florence Nightingale Foundation, London, p. 24.

Fenwick, B. (1889) Medicine and nursing. *Nursing record.* (No number) 2115.

The Medical Act 1944. Pretoria Government Printer.

Nothard, C.A. (1951) Statement on the need of research to C. Searle. Pretoria. April.

The Nursing Act 1944. Pretoria Government Printer.

The Pharmacy Act 1944. Pretoria Government Printer.

SA Nursing Association, 1984, National Nursing Research Register Vol. I Nos. 84/9; 84/10; 84/11; 84/12; 84/13; 84/14 – 84/19; 84/21; 84/31; 84/32; 84/33; 84/34; 84/35; 84/36; 84/40; 84/61; 84/64; 84/83; 84/84; 84/86; 84/90; 84/102; 84/106; 84/109; 84/112; 84/118; 84/119; 84/120; 84/127; 84/128; 84/129; 84/130; 84/131; 84/147; 84/150; 84/156; 84/160; 84/165; 84/190; 84/191; 84/192; 84/196; 84/199; 84/247; 84/248; 84/249; 84/250; 84/251; 84/253; 84/254; 84/258; 84/260; 84/275; 84/276; 84/277; 84/279; 84/280; 84/283; 84/288; 84/305; 84/309; 84/310; 84/313; 84/314; 84/315; 84/319; 84/321; 84/323; 84/326; 84/339; 84/340; 84/341; 84/343 and 84/344.

SA Nursing Association 1984 to 1988. National Nursing Research Registers Vols. I–V. Pretoria.

SA Trained Nurses' Association (1943a) Memorandum to the Minister of Welfare and Demobilization on The Nursing Bill. May.

SA Trained Nurses' Association (1943b) Interview with the Honourable, The Minister of Welfare and Demobilization, Cape Town. May.

Searle, C. (1951) *The problem of the shortage of nursing personnel in Transvaal Public Hospitals.* MA (Soc) Dissertation. University of Pretoria.

Searle, C. (1965) *The History of Nursing in South Africa – a Social Historical Survey.* Struik, Cape Town.

Searle, C. (1986) *Professional Practice: A South African Perspective.* Butterworths, Durban.

Searle, C. (1987) *Ethos of Nursing and Midwifery: A General Perspective.* Butterworths, Durban and Guildford.

# CHAPTER FOURTEEN

# Priorities in nursing research: change and continuity

*Rebecca Bergman*

Research, which is essential to the development of the nursing profession requires a broad, comprehensive approach. It should examine current problems, study basic long-term issues and relate them to past trends. This perspective can facilitate reordering and setting new priorities in the research endeavour.

Styles (1984) described five sequential steps in the development of a profession. Research is the cornerstone on which additional building blocks are added. All five stages are concerned with the knowledge, skills and values of the profession:

generation of knowledge, skills and values through research
transmission through education
authorization through credentialling
mobilization and representation by organization
application of the knowledge, skills and values in practice.

Following Styles' concept of the interaction and mutuality of research with the four other aspects of nursing, I would like to submit three major goals for nursing research:

1. Study, analyse and enhance the *body of knowledge* needed by nursing education and practice in the light of scientific progress and social change;
2. Examine *current education and practice* for quality, effectiveness and efficiency; recommended steps for improvement, and follow-up the results of such action;
3. Study the *mission*, roles and personal meaning of nursing in order to give direction to the profession, reinforce a positive self-perception and public image of the nurse.

These goals should relate to four basic components in nursing:

1.  human – patients, families, nurses, co-workers
2.  health – at all levels along the life span
3.  environment – for healthy living, recovery and peaceful death
4.  health care system – policy, facilities, delivery of care.

The proposed goals are very broad, with many research questions within each goal. Priorities must therefore be set in terms of specific topics and the scope of each research project. A review of the major research areas which were given priority in the past and evaluation of what they achieved, should help direct us to present and future work. We should ask ourselves if some of the priorities in the past fulfilled their purpose and then disappeared from the scene. Did some of the priorities become an integral part of nursing research that need continued study and therefore still remain a priority today? Have other priorities from the past once again become a priority, albeit with a 'new look'?

Let us look at a model depicting the sequence of priorities and challenges in nursing research from mid-century to the present, and see if there are some of the answers to the above questions. I will present the priorities of each stage, and discuss their relevance over time and their importance in today's world.

This model of the development of nursing research starts with the 1940s when nursing research gained impetus, to a large degree due to the growth of university education for nursing in the USA. The model reviews priorities over time, as I perceive them, in relation to three inter-related aspects: content, method and logistics or support systems. Five stages have been delineated in order to emphasize the major priority, but they overlap and indeed there were also other priorities in each stage. In addition to the time dimension, there is also a space dimension in the model with nursing research moving from studies focusing on the local scene, to regional/national and on to international cross-cultural networking.

Stage I focused on the 'who' of nursing, or 'counting heads'. Who are the nurses? Where are they working? What are their demographic characteristics? Who are the applicants to nursing? Which candidates complete the educational program? Who remains in nursing? The methodology was largely descriptive, employing epidemiological sampling and statistical analysis that are today considered rather simplistic.

The major logistic priority was to recruit and prepare nurses to conduct research. Nurses who had completed a master's degree thesis and later those who had successfully gone through the experience of a doctoral dissertation were the main source of qualified manpower for nursing research. The first generation of nurse doctorates were mostly administrators who had earned a Doctor of Education degree. They were followed by PhDs in the basic sciences, with no nursing content. The 1960s saw the first nurse-scientists, who studied basic sciences with a minor in nursing.

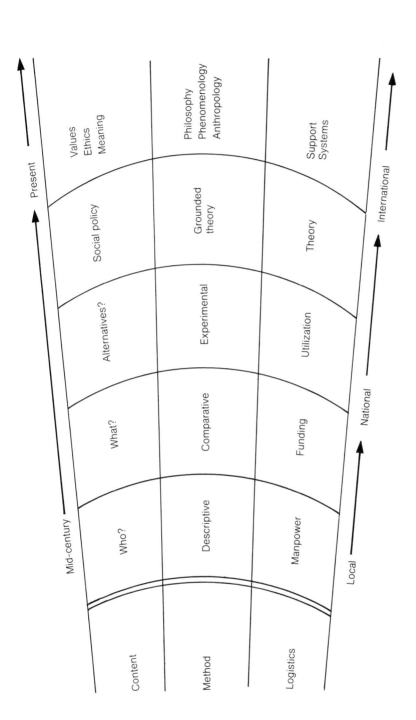

**Figure 14.1** Development of nursing research: content, method and logistic concerns.

The past decade produced the first doctorates in nursing science, with a major in nursing with a cognate in basic science or the humanities (Matarazzo and Abdallah, 1971). The research content carried out by each generation of doctoral students and graduates reflected the focus of their studies.

Knowledge derived from the 'who' studies documented the reservoir of nurse power upon which health care programs could be built. It also revealed the gaps in quantity and quality of nursing personnel to be corrected by the nursing education system. Correction of maldistribution of nurses was undertaken by the socio-economic organizational forces.

I believe that the 'who' of nursing research is an on-going priority. The authors from New Zealand have traced the manpower studies over the past 20 years that responded to needs in the service system. The present emphasis on primary health care requires that the well-qualified generalist nurses move from institutional care to community services, and this redistribution needs to be monitored by research.

From the 1950s research began on requirements for nursing care. In Chapter 11 Bennett describes the development of patient dependency studies in Australia which today serve as a basis for determining staffing needs.

Another important aspect of the 'who' priority is concern about entrants to the profession. Nursing in the western world is today experiencing an acute shortage of applicants to nursing, as evidenced by the professional literature. The predicted demographic drop in the 18–20 year age group is upon us. Further, available candidates in this decade have a much wider career choice than those in earlier periods, with medicine, law, business, engineering and other prestigious and lucrative professions competing for the best candidates. In the USA, 83 000 RNs graduated in 1985, while only 69 000 are expected to complete their basic nursing studies in 1995 (National League for Nursing, 1985) – a drop of 20% in a 10-year period, when there is a growing demand for nurses.

If we hope to fulfil our mission, we need to enlarge the supply of knowledgeable, dedicated nurses. Research must urgently examine the problem of low recruitment, identify its causes in relation to specific situations, in order to have hard data to deal with this critical issue. Issues related to nursing education appear in Chapters 4 to 7. Flaherty (Canada) focuses on preparation of nurse researchers, while the authors from Jamaica, Spain and Brazil relate to education for primary health care in different socio-political settings.

The second stage overlaps with the first, with added depth. It moved from counting heads (who?) to 'what' are the nurses doing. The concern in this period was for optimum utilization of nursing time and energy. This was the heyday of team nursing, so it was necessary to differentiate between the type of care provided by the different levels of nursing personnel. Another aspect was the use of nursing personnel as factotums filling gaps for secretaries, maids, messengers, etc. Time and activity studies were a major priority. They produced data of improper and wasteful use of nurses that shocked both nurses and their employers and resulted in considerable reorganization of personnel and new job descriptions. However, as these lengthy and expensive studies produced similar results time and again in different settings, they were discontinued after a number of years. Today we still need to look at 'what', but in terms of content rather than tasks; for example, developing client independence, patient advocacy and health education.

In this stage the methodology was primarily epidemiological with comparative designs.

The 'what' research, because of its economic implications, was acceptable to agencies and grew in volume. With increased research, the needs for funding become more urgent. Nurses and employers began to look for funds from foundations and government. This 'money' logistic is still present in increasing dimensions. In some countries it has been partially resolved by the establishment of national nursing research institutes which both conduct their own studies and fund outside research. One such example is the British Nursing Research Unit in the Department of Health and Social Security, which has a system of funding regional nursing research centres, guiding local studies, and developing research skills among practitioners.

The third stage of the model is the 'how' period with the focus on clinical practice as differentiated from administration and education in the earlier stages. How are we 'doing' nursing? Are there alternatives to present practice? Are these alternatives safe, ethical, more efficient, more effective, and acceptable to the patient? Some of the earlier studies examined day-to-day routines, e.g. reliability of measuring temperatures, alternative methods of preventing and treating bedsores, handwashing techniques. As clinical specialists with advanced preparation entered the field, research expanded into more specialized subjects such as conservation of energy of acute cardiac patients, feeding very low birth weight infants, or methods to control long-term pain. Today, clinical nursing research continues to be a priority – particularly in relation to the expanding role of the nurse. Intensive care nursing has raised a multitude of nursing questions. The central role of the nurse in long-term care has challenged many researchers. For example, Astrid Norberg in the past several years has produced extremely important findings on the effective and instrumental aspects of feeding the demented (Athlin and Norberg, 1987). This subject is further developed by Norberg in Chapter 9. Aspects of chronicity and nursing research appear in Chapter 8 by Hirschfeld and Krulik. Copp (Chapter 10) reports on research on a major clinical problem – pain control.

Experimental design, which had previously been used in testing educational programs and administrative patterns, was now used in clinical nursing. As controlled clinical research with human subjects raised many ethical and practical problems, nurses often favoured quasi-experimental designs.

The nature of clinical nursing research, which sought ways to improve nursing care, was reflected in the emphasis on logistic dimension. Both researchers and practitioners were anxious to translate the findings into action. Dissemination of reports, their examination, utilization and follow-up received growing attention. Journals devoted to nursing research flourished, as did clinical speciality publications that included research articles. This research interest was also demonstrated by the increasing scope of journal clubs, workshops and research conferences.

Priorities in the fourth stage show a growing concern for social issues. This is the decade during which the 'Health for All by the Year 2000' concept was nurtured, and culminated in the Declaration of Alma-Ata signed by 137 nations in 1978. It was also the quadrennium in which the ICN president declared that the promotion of primary health care would be a major objective of nurses worldwide. Nurses felt the time had come to be a much more aggressive partner in health and welfare decision-making at all levels. They were concerned with social policy of governments and agencies and with social support systems within the community. Nurse researchers, as an arm of the nursing profession, gave attention to these issues.

Angerami (Chapter 7) highlights the socio–political–economic factors involved in establishing primary health care services in Brazil, and the active role played by nursing research is truly exciting. Searle (Chapter 13) traces the political battle of nurses to attain professional status and partnership in policy making in South Africa.

Golander (1988) studied the social support system within a skilled nursing home, and described the importance of the patients' relationships with staff, families and the outer world. Krulik and Hirschfeld (1987) researched families with severe chronically ill aged or children at home. They found that community social support was a major element in the ability of families to cope with such long-term devastating situations.

For many researchers, grounded theory was the method of choice. It permitted inductive analysis of data gathered directly from the target populations. It provided a real-life basis for the hypotheses and theories which grew out of the studies.

Nurse researchers had been using theoretical frameworks in many studies, but from the 1970s much greater emphasis was placed on this aspect, particularly in research required for academic degrees. Nursing theory began to flourish – books by theorists on their own work, as well as texts analysing nursing theories and theory development appeared on the market. Nurse researchers can learn much from theories of nursing and those of other disciplines. They would also do well to be open-minded, and see these theories as guides to reflection rather than as a definitive frame to be religiously adhered to. The use of established theories, as well as the development of new conceptual frameworks are well illustrated in the chapter on pain (Chapter 10).

The fifth stage, that we are now experiencing, has a new emphasis – the meaning of nursing, values and ethics. Such questions have been discussed since Florence Nightingale, but more recently nurses are seeking answers through research. Evaluative studies are looking not only to efficiency and effectiveness of care, but to the quality of life of patients. The affective aspects of nursing for the patient and family, as well as for the nurse herself (satisfaction, stress, self-actualization, autonomy) are among the major topics. Ethical codes and guidelines are being supplemented by studies on ethical decision-making. An Israeli doctoral student is now completing her dissertation on how and why nurses respond to ethical dilemmas in the hospital. Watson's theory of caring, is being applied and examined in relation to various age groups and clinical conditions by a number of researchers. The essence of her approach can be seen in her description of the contrast between the traditional and the caring model; the caring model being much more respecting of the individual, affective in nature, and based on a deeper personal involvement (Watson, 1985).

Methodology in this type of research utilizes philosophical, phenomenological, and anthropological approaches. Meleis (1985) calls this the 'perceived view' in contrast to the 'received view' (scientific method). 'Significant holistic problems in nursing have been ignored because they are neither reducible, quantifiable, nor objective.... The perceived view incorporates ideas that are subjective, intuitive, humanistic.'

The development of nursing research, conducting sophisticated in-depth studies as an integral part of nursing practice, has led to the need to institutionalize a support system for nursing research.

On the international level, the International Council of Nurses and the World Health Organization are important sources for research policy. ICN (1984) prepared a directory of nursing research units based on data gathered with the help of the National Nurses' Associations. They identified 33 research units, of which 22 were in the USA, two in Canada, eight in Europe and one in New Zealand.

Farrell and Christensen in Chapter 2 present the cross-national nursing research in the WHO European Region.

On the national level, in 1983, the US House of Representatives proposed the Institute of Nursing within the National Institutes of Health – which is described in Chapter 3 by Hinshaw and Heinrich. The United Kingdom national nursing research system was previously mentioned.

Dienemann (1987), in a survey of 124 US graduate nursing programs, found 50 nursing research centres. She concluded that the presence of such centres 'contributes to research productivity within the profession.' The centres centralize research resources, teach research, sponsor conferences, create a research climate, publish research findings, offer consultation to faculty, and co-ordinate research activities.

In her comprehensive book on clinical nursing research, Lieska (1986) depicted the internal and external networking of nursing research for nursing practice. Internally, the nurse researcher interacts with staff and students, professional mentors and supervisors, and with other nurse specialists and disciplines in the institution. Externally her contacts are other agencies, consultants, universities, consortia and professional organizations.

A further concern, in our present stage of research, is to gain equal access to the interdisciplinary forums and research foundations. To achieve this, nursing must present proposals for funding that compete favourably with other submissions. Nursing research articles published in refereed journals must meet appropriate standards and be presented in a scholarly manner. The credibility and status of nursing research will stand or fall with the kind of work we produce.

The above review of priorities in nursing research over the past half century shows that most of the priorities, in a comprehensive perspective, continue to be important today. The emphases and specifics have changed and will continue to change in order to respond to scientific and social change in our world.

It is the responsibility of the nursing profession, through its researchers and leadership, to identify needed research, set priorities, carry out the studies and disseminate the findings for implementation in practice, education and organization. Hopefully, this book which brings together various foci of nursing research in different parts of the world, will contribute to the growth and impact of meaningful international nursing research.

## REFERENCES

Athlin, E. and Norberg, A. (1987) Caregivers' attitudes to and interpretations of the behavior of severely demented patients during feeding in a patient assignment care system. *Int. J. Nurs. Stud.*, **24** (2), 145–154.

Dienemann, J. (1987) Nursing Research Centers. *Int. J. Nurs. Stud.*, **24** (1). 35–44.

Golander, H. (1988) Under the guise of passivity. *J. Adv. Nurs.*, **13** (2), 26–31.

International Council of Nurses (1984) *Directory of Nursing Research Units.* International Council of Nurses, Geneva.

Krulik, T. and Hirschfeld, M. (1987) *Caregivers of severely handicapped children and aged at home.* Tel Aviv University, Tel Aviv.

Lieska, A. (ed.) (1986) *Clinical Nursing Research.* Aspen publications, Rockville, Md.

Matarazzo, J. and Abdallah, F. (1971) Doctoral education of nurses in the United States. *Nurs. Res.*, **20**, 404–413.

Meleis, A. (1985) *Theoretical Nursing: Development and Progress.* Lippincott, Philadelphia.

National League for Nursing (1985) *Nursing Data Review.* National League for Nursing, New York.

Styles, M. (1984) Lecture given at Tel Aviv University.

Watson, J. (1985) *Nursing: Human science and human care.* Appleton-Century-Crofts, New York.

# Index